BLOOD WORK

THE LEWIS HENRY MORGAN LECTURES
presented at the University of Rochester
Rochester, New York

JANET CARSTEN

BLOOD WORK

Life and Laboratories in Penang

FOREWORD BY THOMAS GIBSON

DUKE UNIVERSITY PRESS

Durham and London

2019

© 2019 Duke University Press
All rights reserved
Printed and bound by CPI Group (UK) Ltd, Croydon, CR0 4YY
Designed by Matthew Tauch
Typeset in Arno Pro by Westchester Publishing Services

Library of Congress Cataloging-in-Publication Data

Names: Carsten, Janet, author.
Title: Blood work : life and laboratories in Penang /
Janet Carsten.
Description: Durham : Duke University Press, 2019. |
Series: The Lewis Henry Morgan lectures | Includes
bibliographical references and index.
Identifiers: LCCN 2018061081 (print)
LCCN 2019005934 (ebook)
ISBN 9781478005698 (ebook)
ISBN 9781478004202 (hardcover : alk. paper)
ISBN 9781478004813 (pbk. : alk. paper)
Subjects: LCSH: Blood—Symbolic aspects. | Blood—Social
aspects—Malaysia—Pulau Pinang (State) | Blood—
Religious aspects. | Blood—Collection and preservation—
Malaysia—Pulau Pinang (State) | Blood donors—Malaysia—
Pulau Pinang (State)
Classification: LCC GT498.B55 (ebook) | LCC GT498.B55 C37
2019 (print) | DDC 306.4—dc23
LC record available at https://lccn.loc.gov/2018061081

Cover art: Slides arranged on a lab bench for manual blood grouping
(detail). Photo by the author.

IN MEMORY OF SALLY LAIRD,
1956–2010

CONTENTS

The Lewis Henry Morgan Lectures were originally conceived in 1961 by Bernard Cohn, who was then chair of the Department of Anthropology and Sociology at the University of Rochester. A founder of modern cultural anthropology, Morgan was one of Rochester's most famous intellectual figures and a patron of the university; he left a substantial bequest to the university for the founding of a women's college. The lectures named in his honor have now been presented annually for over fifty years and constitute the longest-running such series in North America. Morgan's monograph *Systems of Consanguinity and Affinity*, published in 1871, inaugurated the systematic cross-cultural study of kinship. Morgan's other two main areas of interest concerned the ethnography of Native North America, *The League of the Ho-dé-no-sau-nee or Iroquois* (1851), and the comparative study of civilizations, *Ancient Society* (1881).

It was to explore the way these interests had been developed by the discipline of anthropology over the subsequent decades that the first three Morgan Lecturers were selected. Meyer Fortes delivered the first full set of Morgan Lectures in 1963, which resulted in his monograph *Kinship and the Social Order* (1969). This was followed by lectures by Fred Eggan on Native North America in 1964, which resulted in his monograph *The American Indian: Perspectives for the Study of Social Change* (1966), and by Robert Adams on ancient Mesopotamia and Mexico in 1964, which resulted in his monograph *The Evolution of Urban Society* (1966).

As the fiftieth anniversary of the first Morgan Lectures approached, the Department of Anthropology decided to invite a series of three lecturers to speak on the same set of topics as the first three. In 2011, Professor Marisol de la Cadena delivered the annual lecture on the subject of indigenous politics in the Andes. In 2013, Professor Peter van der Veer delivered the annual lecture on contemporary understandings of the value of comparison. The present volume is based on the Lewis Henry Morgan Lecture that Professor Janet Carsten delivered at the University of Rochester on November 7, 2012, and the workshop held the following day. The formal discussants at the workshop included Eleana Kim and Sherine Hamdy, both now at the University of California, Irvine; and Ayala Emmett and Ann Russ, both at the University of Rochester.

Professor Carsten's monograph illustrates many of the transformations that the study of kinship has undergone over the past fifty years. Her research on the fluid meanings of blood in the highly technical and modern setting of Malaysian hospitals combines the concern of classical British social anthropology with kinship as a form of morality; of American cultural anthropology with kinship as a domain of symbols and meanings that are particular to each culture; and of science and technology studies with the processes by which modern societies attempt to purify social life into the separate domains of kinship, politics, economics, science, and religion.

By following the meanings of a single natural symbol as it flows from one "domain" to another, Carsten is able to call into question many assumptions that have guided social research in Malaysia. As she points out, most researchers focus on one or another of Malaysia's ethnic groups, which include the Muslim Malays, the predominantly Buddhist Chinese, and the predominantly Hindu Indians. This overlap between "race" and religion, and the way these categories are reproduced in an essentialized way by government policy and the media, makes it all too easy for the social analyst to accept these categories uncritically when conducting research.

In fact, very many—and possibly most—urban Malaysians work alongside members of other ethnicities on a daily basis, and the degree to which they have come to share similar sets of attitudes and values is a matter to be determined empirically. This is the methodological advantage of following a symbolically charged substance like blood as it flows from one body through a multicultural techno-sociological apparatus into other bodies. Each ethnic group has its own particular practices regarding the preparation, sharing, and consumption of food; rules relating to kinship, marriage, and childbirth; and long-standing political values and affiliations. Despite this sociocultural pluralism, everyone regards blood as a substance derived from individuals who have their own reasons for donating blood and as a substance that can give life to any member of the whole human community.

Carsten concludes by arguing that the social and affective relations that are formed between coworkers of diverse ethnic backgrounds in even the most sterile laboratory environments are a necessary condition for the successful functioning of the Malaysian medical system as an integrated whole. More generally, she shows how the sharing of blood with the community at large is one of the ways in which Malaysia has become a modern nation whose citizens perceive themselves to be related to each other partly through idioms of kinship and family. In Malay terms, being *saudara* (kin) is derived from being of one blood—*satu* (one) and *darah* (blood)— according to at least some of her interlocutors' etymology of a Malay term for siblingship that is often used for kinship in general.

It is a testament to the fluidity of the meanings of blood and kinship that an alternative etymology of saudara derives the term from the Sanskrit words *saha-* (together) and *udara* (womb), meaning uterine sibling. Following this etymology would lead us away from the concept of kinship as the sharing of a common substance and toward the concept of kinship as a form of sociality derived from the sharing of a common space such as a womb, a house, or a tomb, a notion that is found widely throughout the Austronesian language area. But as Carsten demonstrated in her earlier work on Malay kinship in a rural village on the island of Langkawi, *The Heat of the Hearth* (1997), there is no necessary conflict between these two meanings of *saudara*. Blood is held to be derived from the transformation of food, particularly breast milk and rice, and so the shared blood of kinship can be acquired through commensality within a shared domestic space. Similarly, in urban Malaysia, and perhaps in many other ethnically plural societies, the acquisition of a shared sense of national identity may occur through commensality and other forms of sociality within a shared workplace. It is one of the great merits of this monograph that it directs our attention to the way these micro-sociological interactions form the basis on which macro-sociological forms of solidarity such as shared national cultures may be either generated or undermined.

THOMAS GIBSON

Editor, Lewis Henry Morgan Monograph Series (2007–2013)

July 2018

ACKNOWLEDGMENTS

Writing and researching this book has been a process of serious debt accumulation. I am all too conscious of the many acts of unexpected kindness and generosity on the part of individuals and institutions that have made this work possible, and the many productive insights and comments from those who listened to or read earlier versions of this work. I am conscious too of the remaining flaws—which I claim as my own.

I am deeply grateful to the Leverhulme Trust, whose generous award of a Major Research Fellowship enabled me to carry out the research and to write over a three-year period from 2007 to 2010. Without that support, this work could not have been accomplished. I also thank the British Academy for a Small Research Grant that made a vital contribution to fieldwork expenses.

In Penang I owe an enormous debt to Khoo Salma Nasution for introducing me to doctors and for helping to facilitate the beginning of this research. She and Abdur-Razzaq Lubis provided their unique depth of knowledge of Penang and hospitable support throughout my research. I am extremely grateful to Professor Dr. Nor Hafizah Selamat for her assistance in providing local sponsorship for the research, and to her and Professor Dato' Dr. Rashidah Shuib for offering affiliation to KANITA at Universiti Sains Malaysia. Dato' Dr. Hjh Wazir Jahan Begum Karim and Dato' Dr. Hj. Mohd Razha Rashid provided intellectual sustenance, warm hospitality, and the benefits of long friendship to me and to my family during visits to Penang. In Penang and Kuala Lumpur, Dr. Yeoh Seng Guan gave his generous advice and helpful contacts as well as reading and commenting on draft chapters.

I am very grateful to the Economic Planning Unit (EPU) of the Prime Minister's Department of the government of Malaysia and the State Government of Penang for permission to carry out the research.

The hospitals, doctors, and staff of clinical pathology labs and blood banks that are the subject of this book have been anonymized for reasons of confidentiality. I was welcomed with unfailing friendliness by staff in the hospitals where I carried out research, and was granted unique access to the spaces that I describe. I have no adequate words to thank those who answered my many questions and tolerated my presence with unfailing patience and good humor. I hope I have done justice here to their integrity, commitment, and hard work.

An earlier version of chapter 4 was previously published under the title "Ghosts, Commensality, and Scuba Diving: Tracing Kinship and Sociality in Clinical Pathology Labs and Blood Banks in Penang" in *Vital Relations: Modernity and the Persistent Life of Kinship*, edited by Susan McKinnon and Fenella Cannell (School for Advanced Research Press, 2013). Some material in chapter 3 appeared in an earlier form in an article titled "'Searching for the Truth': Tracing the Moral Properties of Blood in Malaysian Clinical Pathology Labs" in *Blood Will Out: Essays on Liquid Transfers and Flows*, special issue of the *Journal of the Royal Anthropological Institute* 19 (May 2013). I am grateful to the editors and publishers and to the Royal Anthropological Institute of Great Britain and Ireland for permission to use this material here.

It is a special blessing to have worked for many years in the most collegial, friendly, and intellectually stimulating setting. My colleagues and students in social anthropology at the University of Edinburgh have been unfailingly supportive and constructive at every stage of research and writing. I owe a particular debt to Richard Baxstrom, Ian Harper, Toby Kelly, and Rebecca Marsland for their encouragement and productive comments on early drafts of chapters at meetings of a small writing group in 2009–10. Jacob Copeman contributed his intellectual enthusiasm and expertise on blood on numerous occasions. Resto Cruz provided invaluable assistance at the final stage of manuscript submission.

The invitation to deliver a Morgan Lecture at the University of Rochester in 2012 and the accompanying workshop provided a wonderful and unlooked-for opportunity to discuss draft chapters and the material on which they are based. I am deeply grateful to Tom Gibson, Bob Foster, Ayala Emmett, Eleana Kim, Sherine Hamdy, Ann Russ, and other participants at the workshop, and to members of the Department of Anthropology at Rochester for their outstanding hospitality and productive comments.

The anonymous readers of the manuscript for Duke University Press were exceptionally generous and stimulating in their suggestions—many of which have been silently incorporated. I owe a huge debt to them and to Ken Wissoker for their enthusiasm and constructive interventions.

Papers based on material in this book have been given at seminars and invited lectures at Aarhus University; Goldsmiths University of London; Helsinki University; the London School of Economics; the National University of Singapore; New York University; the University of California, Berkeley; the University of Cambridge; the University of Edinburgh; the University of Malaya; the University of Manchester; the University of Michigan; Universiti Sains Malaysia; the University of Toronto; and the University of Virginia; and at a conference titled "The Difference Kinship Makes" at the School for Advanced Research in Santa Fe. I am very grateful to audiences and participants at all these places for their suggestions and comments.

Sophie Day has been a close listener and a source of creative ideas and warm friendship over many years—I am more grateful for these than I can say. I am deeply indebted to Veena Das, Gillian Feeley-Harnik, Sarah Franklin, Emily Martin, Susan McKinnon, Rayna Rapp, and Kath Weston for the inspiration their work has provided and for their productive comments at different junctures.

Sally Laird brought the remarkable qualities of her intelligence to bear on the first stories from this research, as she did to so much else. In urging me to keep in view the patients' side of the experiences I have described, she provided a salutary reminder of what is at stake in blood work. The most loving and generous of friends, she saw clearly into the life of things.

Finally, I owe my deepest gratitude to Jessica Spencer and Jonathan Spencer for providing a sustaining blend of familial, culinary, and intellectual support over the years of research and writing—as well as in its interruptions. Jessica lived with me in Penang for seven months in 2008. During that time and since, she has contributed questions and insights about blood, as well as much else, in a spirit of generosity, humor, perceptiveness, and loyalty that is uniquely her own. Jonathan has accompanied me on the intellectual journey, paid extended visits to Penang, and been a source of wise advice and unstinting support at every stage. In reading the manuscript of this book and giving me the benefit of his acute and creative editorial skills, he has—as always—gone beyond what might reasonably be expected.

In the modern world, the Indian Ocean's cosmopolitanism was messy and inconsistent, and often it shattered under pressure. It developed as a cultural response to the demands of living in a world of strangers; its archive lies in popular culture, in the unwritten conventions of urban sociability, and in the shape of the landscape as much as in the writing of poets and visionaries.
—SUNIL S. AMRITH, *Crossing the Bay of Bengal*

No one knows why some individuals experience "pump-head": a disturbance of mood and cognition brought on by having your blood moved beyond the confines of the body, but a charge nurse in a cardiothoracic intensive care unit told me that up to a third of her patients experience it. Many are violent as they come round; security guards have to hold them down as they are sedated with powerful antipsychotic medication. Some are merely quiet, "not themselves." . . . Some become inappropriate and disinhibited.
—GAVIN FRANCIS, *Adventures in Human Being*

When I arrive in the operating theatre, about 15 people are already present—the anaesthetised patient on an operating table, the surgical nurses quietly harvesting veins from the patient's legs, as well as several other nurses and a group of nursing students observing surgery from the vantage point of a low platform near the head of the patient. Also present are three staff trained in cardiovascular perfusion (operating the heart-lung machine) and two anaesthetists. Pleasant music is playing in the background. The cardiac surgeon, Dr Ho, greets me with a courteous "Welcome, Prof," and I thank him for allowing me to observe that morning's triple bypass surgery. Once the vein harvesting is completed, the patient is ready for surgery.

The heart-lung machine is being set up. Attached to the pump are masses of long transparent tubes, which connect to the tank. As they set up the machine, the medical perfusionists repeatedly tap different sections of tubes to make sure no air bubbles are trapped that might cause a fatal embolism. A point of high tension occurs when they transfer the patient from his own heart to the machine—it proceeds a bit like a rocket launch with a synchronised countdown and different tasks accurately coordinated. All goes well.

At the centre of the operating theatre everything is quiet and very concentrated—except when Dr Ho throws out a question to me, to the student nurses, to the perfusionist, or the anaesthetist. Outside this quiet centre, on the periphery of activities, there is a more relaxed atmosphere. A nursing auxiliary shows photos from a recent excursion up Penang Hill. In the lulls when he is not checking the heart-lung machine and its readings, the supervisor of medical perfusion jokes around, at one point conducting a fantasy orchestra. Anaesthetists and others come and go.

From time to time as the operation proceeds, Dr Ho asks the student nurses questions: "What do we call this?" (Answer, pericardium.) "What does this do?" Mainly, they fail to answer.

Dr Ho makes sure I get to see the live heart beating before bypass. The patient's head and neck are covered by green surgical sheets. One of the perfusionists tells me that the patient is divided into a sterile zone— where they are operating—and a non-sterile zone under covers. The result of this is that the patient doesn't appear like a live person at all. The skin of his legs looks waxy and inert, perhaps partly because of the lights—a bit like an anatomical model.

Dr Ho hardly appears to communicate with the surgical nurses by micro-signs; they seem to know what to do without being told. Instructions to the anaesthetist and the medical perfusionist are issued in a more ritualised fashion and then repeated back: "Pump down." "Pump down, Dr Ho," and suchlike. He teases the young perfusionist that the patient's life is in her hands—she is the most important person there.

At one point Dr Ho pauses to ask the student nurses, "How do we know this patient is alive?" No one answers. A moment passes before

Dr Ho continues, "The patient is in limbo—cooled to 28 degrees, and the heart is not beating. He is neither alive nor dead. We hope he's alive. But we can't tell till he's taken off the pump."

• • •

This edited extract from my notes of February 2008 was written after one of the more eventful mornings of my fieldwork in Penang. I had not planned to observe cardiac surgery. But I had been invited just that morning to follow the medical perfusionists who worked in the clinical pathology labs and blood banks in one of the hospitals where I was carrying out research—an offer that, after a few seconds' hesitation, seemed impossible to refuse. Medical perfusionists operate the heart-lung machines that are essential to coronary bypass surgery, ensuring the continued transmission of oxygenated blood to the body and the removal of carbon dioxide while the heart is stopped. Dr. Ho's question to the student nurses was a trick one, but it highlights what is indeed a mystery: at this point in surgery there was no way to know whether the patient was alive or dead.

Shigehisa Kuriyama eloquently poses just this question in the closing passages of his wonderful historical exploration of the divergence of classical Greek and Chinese medicine, *The Expressiveness of the Body*:

> What separates the living from the dead?
>
> Life's presence is manifest to the senses, yet ever eludes the reach of our comprehension. We plainly see the metamorphoses of vitality in someone running, stopping, looking back, turning pale; we can hear the supple force of life in the sharpness of precise diction, and in the soft insinuations of tone; we can even grasp vital power with our fingers, here at the wrist, feel it pulsating or flowing. But in the end the mystery persists. (Kuriyama 2002, 271)

Blood, as we learn from Kuriyama's study, and as I show in this book, is at the center of this mystery.[1] What separates the living from the dead? The answer perhaps seems obvious. And yet recent ethnographies from Southeast Asia show all too clearly how reluctantly the dead may leave the living or the living may relinquish their dead. In central Vietnam, Heonik Kwon (2008) has described the remarkably vital and ubiquitous presence that "ghosts of war" continue to exert on the lives of the living more than twenty years after the cessation of hostilities. Evoking fear, humor, grief, or poignancy—and sometimes all of these at once—ghosts here seem just too full of life. In a more domestic and intimate register, in the Philippines, Fenella Cannell (1999) depicts the difficulty that Catholic Bicolanos have in separating after death and the potentially deleterious effects of this reluctance for the health of the living. When "the dead pull the living towards them," further deaths are liable to ensue, and for this reason "the living must resist" (163).

But the subject of this work is not death or rituals of mourning. On the contrary, it is what in many cultures is viewed as the very stuff of life. Blood is not only essential for life, it is also often an idiom of connection between persons. In English, we speak readily of "blood ties" or "blood relatives." The pervasiveness of such idioms makes it hard to focus on them or to subject them to an analytic gaze that might tease apart their resonance and significance, to calibrate the myriad qualities that supposedly "flow in the blood." Anthropologists, like other proper participants in their own cultures, are prone to adopt such locutions as if they were self-evident and without always specifying when they are translating indigenous terms (Carsten 2011, 30; Ingold 2007, 110–11). In the field of kinship studies, anthropologists might be expected to think carefully about the meanings of connections that are articulated in terms of blood, but this is not necessarily so. David Schneider's famous rendering of *American Kinship*, in which relatives are defined by blood, and blood is the symbol of "shared biogenetic material" ([1968] 1980, 25), to take just one example, not only occludes the relation between blood and "biogenetic substance," but it also fails to probe the meanings of blood as a symbol in American culture or to take account of their instability (Carsten 2004, 111–12).

The starting point for this book, however, was not American kinship but a paddy field on the island of Langkawi in Malaysia. There, transplanting rice seedlings one morning with a group of village women in the early 1980s, and up to my calves in water, I had a conversation that has remained vivid over several decades. One of the women noticed me pulling a leech off the back of my leg and the trickle of blood where it came away. This immediately sparked a lively commentary on the nature of my blood—how red it was and how well it flowed, properties that were noted with approval. Over the subsequent months, on and off, there were further conversations about qualities of blood. Blood groups were a topic of particular interest—

Group O was thought to be best because of its universal donor status, and I was surprised by this knowledge. The centrality of blood to kinship and its derivation from food in Malay ideas were a focus of my research. And the very term for kin in Malay, "saudara," is locally described as a contraction of *satu darah*, literally, one blood (see Carsten 1997, ch. 4). But what struck me in that paddy field was the realization that physical properties of blood were a subject of keen speculation and that, in ways that were not necessarily obvious, they connected to its symbolic range and potential.

In what may seem a bizarrely literalist move, the research described in this book was devised to explore the pathways along which blood travels as it moves between different domains of social life—kinship, for example, but also moral or religious ideas and biomedical ones. How do people negotiate between the physical manifestations of blood in everyday workplaces, such as clinical pathology labs, blood banks, or operating rooms, and its metaphorical allusions? What are the connections that enable this flow or the breakpoints that permit seemingly obvious connections to be severed? What properties of blood enhance an efflorescence of potential qualities and resonances? In short, what *is* blood? And what, if anything, could excavating something like a "theory of blood" contribute to our understandings of kinship and wider relatedness—or the persistent mystery, to which I have alluded, of the living and the dead? In planning this research, I hazarded that blood banks and clinical pathology labs might be interesting places to explore these questions. Malaysia, through my research experience and familiarity, was an obvious point of departure; Penang—with its long and complex history of trade, demographic diversity, its confluence of multiple ethnicities and religions, and its abundant medical facilities—seemed to offer particularly rich possibilities.

Like many ethnographies, this work is intended to be both of general and specific interest. It is at once an anthropology of contemporary urban life in Malaysia in multiethnic settings and an analysis of blood as bodily substance and symbol. Although my intellectual starting point has been kinship, this is far from being a conventional work on kinship. Instead, like its subject matter, it resists confinement to a particular domain. I depict aspects of social life in Malaysia, including interactions in the workplace, to illuminate how these are shaped by, and shape, processes of gender, ethnicity, kinship, class, and morality. The lens of blood allows us to observe these social processes in action, paradoxically, by placing them in the background rather than the foreground. I did not set out to study gender, class, or ethnicity in the labs or blood banks; nevertheless, close observation of these spaces may tell us more about creating and erasing social distinctions in Malaysia than if they had been the explicit focus of my inquiries. In following "the social life of blood" in Penang, I have also aimed to understand more generally what blood is and how it works as a powerful and highly plastic symbol. This part of the story is both particular to Malaysia and an aspect of naturalization and domaining processes more broadly. The present chapter begins to explore the nature of blood and sets out the main themes and structure of the book. It also locates the research by introducing its setting in Penang and describing the process of fieldwork.

Blood

What is blood? The central premise of this book is that the answer to this question is not self-evident. Its vital properties encapsulate the mystery of life and death—as my opening vignette suggests. The many meanings attributed to blood are neither knowable in advance nor stable across different historical eras and cultural contexts. What is striking, however, is the power and pervasiveness of blood symbolism in many cultures. Blood has an unusual capacity to evoke relational ties on different scales, to connote life and death, violence, sacrifice, and worth. Blood may denote physiological and social sameness as well as difference and, to a singular degree, its literal or metaphorical presence can elicit strong emotional responses. What gives blood this range of capacities? How does it operate as material substance, sign, and symbol? In the following pages I draw on a diverse anthropological literature to suggest some answers to these questions; the succeeding chapters pursue the argument in specific ethnographic settings.

Any discussion of the remarkable capacities of blood might justifiably begin with its material properties: its striking color, liquidity, warmth while in the body, its smell, and the way it solidifies and changes color when spilled. This nexus of physical characteristics makes blood unique.[2] One does not have to stray far from its physical properties to suggest reasons for blood's capacity to evoke emotional responses (Taylor 1992; Turner 1967). The stopping or spilling of blood whether in illness, by accident, or with intentional acts of violence may literally signal the difference between life or death. Within or beyond the body, too much blood flow or too little quickly have lethal consequences. Blood is bound up with life and death in equal measure.

So much, so obvious, one might think. But sometimes the obviousness of phenomena obstructs our ability to analyze them clearly or prevents us from seeing that there might be something worth probing further. The striking physiological properties of blood and its strong association with life and death are integral to its aptness for metaphorization and its generativity in symbolism. In Leviticus 17:1–15, blood is described as the animating life-force and the bearer of the soul (see also Anidjar 2014, 7). The consumption of blood is proscribed in Judaism and in Islam, and animals to be eaten must be drained of blood when they are slaughtered. The fluidity of blood in a healthy body may readily suggest agentive force, animation, and vitality (see also Feeley-Harnik 1995). Kuriyama shows how "in Chinese medicine, blood and *qi* [breath] were essentially the same." They were "complementary facets of a unique vitality" (2002, 229).[3] In chapter 1 we will see that associations between blood and life are crucial in motivating donors in Penang to give blood. "Give blood; save a life" is a slogan used in donation campaigns that has wide public resonance. But the links between blood and life may also strike a chord with medical lab technologists. This may be marked in literal, material, and scientific terms by medical lab technologists as they go about the mundane tasks of analyzing and recording diagnostic test results or screening donated blood, as described in chapter 3. But such connections may also be evoked in more metaphysical ways when lab staff articulate the risks of their workplace, consider the importance of test results for patients, ponder the question of whether blood itself is alive, or discuss the possible presence of ghosts in the labs—as we learn in chapter 4.

An important contention of this book is that the unspoken elisions between these different ways of speaking about blood encapsulate not only the polyvalence of blood but also the way that meanings may be entangled with each other so that a reference in one register may carry the possibility of evoking responses in another. Blood is in many cultures a reservoir of familial, religious, and political symbolic meanings. In his exploration of blood and Christianity, Gil Anidjar refers to "the wide sanguification of rhetoric" (2014, 7). As anthropologists, how can we elucidate what enables such a flow of meanings between supposedly separate domains? Can we render these processes visible and unpick their political salience? In the sections drawn from newspaper accounts that precede each of the main ethnographic chapters, I trace some of the resonances of blood in public media in Malaysia at the time of my research. The section that precedes chapter 3 describes how, at a highly fraught moment in Malaysian political life, a contested blood sample of the leader of the opposition, Anwar Ibrahim, was deemed to have the capacity to "reveal the truth" about his moral character. The extraordinary political showdown that climaxed with Anwar's arrest in July 2008 on a charge of sodomy continued to play out for several years and resulted in his eventual imprisonment (see Allers 2013; Trowell 2015).

Blood's literal capacity to flow, often associated with health and vigor, thus has metaphorical counterparts. In an earlier essay (Carsten 2011), I suggested that we might compare this propensity to the attributes of money and ghosts, which likewise tend to move between different spheres in apparently unconstrained ways. But there are areas to which neither money nor ghosts should have access. Ghosts of course are normally kept at bay from everyday life. Love and money are, in Western contexts, often claimed to be mutually antithetical (see Bloch and Parry 1989). Not unconnectedly, Richard Titmuss ([1970] 1997) famously argued that payment for blood donation put the safety of blood transfusion services at risk. Without undermining his pioneering insights, this book suggests that payment for donation captures only one small part of the risks to which donated blood is potentially vulnerable. It is the uncontainability of blood, its simultaneous permeability in multiple fields, that makes it so difficult to safeguard its security from contamination—as recent blood scandals in several countries have demonstrated.[4] Efforts intended to ensure the safety of blood, by preempting certain categories of people from donating, reinforce social exclusions and are thus prone to create further ricochets of resonance between different meanings of blood.[5]

In thinking through blood's unusual characteristics, I have found a helpful entry point in Geoffrey C. Bowker and Susan Leigh Star's (1999) discussion of "boundary objects"—objects that "can inhabit multiple contexts at once, and have both local and shared meaning" (293). Pertinently for this study, Star uses the term "boundary objects" to consider the ways in which scientists navigate different meanings (Star 1989; Star and Griesemer 1989) but argues that the term is not restricted to scientific contexts (Bowker and Star 1999, 297). Boundary objects "have different meanings in different social worlds but their structure is common enough to more than one world to make them recognizable, a means of translation. The creation and management of boundary objects is a key process in developing and maintaining coherence across intersecting communities" (Bowker and Star 1999, 297).

Scientific work, as Bowker and Star note, is composed of different communities of practice and different viewpoints—they mention lab technicians and janitors (1999, 296). The scope of the current study includes blood donors, medical lab technologists and other lab workers, patients, and the relatives of people in these categories, as well as clinicians and others. It thus extends well beyond the realms of scientific practice, and this suggests that the idea of the boundary object might prove insufficient for the contexts described here.

In chapter 1, I consider the form that blood donors in Penang complete prior to donation as a kind of boundary object. The donor form is an important means by which blood, and the donors from whom it is sourced, is categorized. But I also ask whether the concept of boundary object could apply to blood itself. What would it mean to think of blood in this way? If such an attempt seems to indicate limitations to the idea of the boundary object, Bowker and Star's attentiveness to processes of naturalization in the work of classification simultaneously suggests the possible analytic purchase of their concept. Blood's unusual properties, I argue below, are strongly linked to its naturalizing capacities. Before turning to naturalization, however, another dimension of blood's pervasive resonance is pertinent: temporality.

Probing the extraordinary polyvalence of blood, Kath Weston (2013) has shown how metaphors of blood that occur in contemporary depictions of the financial system enfold different somatic models with different historicities. Images of "lifeblood," "circulation," "flow," "liquidity," "hemorrhaging," "stagnation," or the necessity of "blood-letting" in the financial system occur alongside each other. While the circulatory model discovered by William Harvey in the early seventeenth century is predominant here, Weston elucidates how older notions that predate Harvey's model are also present. In another striking case, Brazilian peasants described by Maya Mayblin (2013) use a modern technique of intravenous rehydration to replenish the fluid in their body when they feel unwell, but in so doing they evoke a Catholic imagery of Christ's sacrifice in which blood, sweat, tears, and water can be seen as transformations of each other and have a particular local ecological and religious salience. In a quite different setting, Jacob Copeman (2013) has described how the importance of the literal use of blood to paint the portraits of Indian martyrs of independence is intended to evoke the past sacrifice of those martyrs and also vividly reminds the viewers of these paintings that their own blood may be called upon in further acts of political sacrifice in the future. In a radically different context, Emily Martin (2013) has depicted how contemporary medical discourses surrounding MRI scans of the brain, from which blood has mysteriously been purged, reveal a deeper archaeology in which different kinds of blood, referring to somatic models with a different historicity, occur in a gendered hierarchy in the body.

In all of these examples, blood evokes understandings that originate in different historical epochs, but these are collapsed and condensed into particular images, locutions, or practices. A similar entanglement of temporalities is suggested in chapter 4, where medical lab technologists move between radically different registers when they refer to the specific results of diagnostic tests in scientific terms but also speak of the "mystery" of blood and its unique capacity to reveal the truth. The unusual truth-bearing quality of blood has been noted in quite different cultural contexts (see Bildhauer 2013; Copeman 2013). Blood, as Copeman (2014, 10) pithily observes, "is a substance that contains its own historicity." And different evocations or imagery of blood may resonate with, or comment on, each other (Copeman 2014, 10).[6] The relational capacities of blood suggest that we should emphasize the plurality of these historicities. Such implicit temporal entanglements both reinforce and complicate the emphasis that David Warren Sabean and Simon Teuscher (2013) have placed on an apparently more straightforward and chronological historical specificity of ideas about blood in European kinship.

Mayblin (2013) has observed that, for the Brazilian peasants she studied, the transubstantiation of wine into the blood of Jesus in the Eucharist is a literal truth, essential to their sense of the beauty of, and aesthetic pleasure in, the Catholic Mass. She notes that a crucial quality of blood is that it can function as both metaphor and metonym—and this is central to theological debates about the Christian Eucharist (see Bynum 2007). In this sense, the link between Christ's sacrifice and the daily sacrifice of labor is made tangible. Metaphorical and material understandings of blood are in constant play with each other, and this is part of blood's heightened capacity for naturalization and its symbolic power. It is as though blood's animation exerts its own force of propulsion, extending in multiple directions from material to metaphorical realms and vice versa.

Drawing attention to this interplay of signification in multiple directions, Weston emphasizes "the generative possibilities of blood, as well as its ability to pre-empt debate as it naturalizes social processes, and perfuses multiple domains" (2013, 33). She uses the term "meta-materiality" (35) to convey that what is invoked goes beyond both metaphor and the material—but also, and simultaneously, relies on both the material and the metaphorical to generate further resonances and further naturalizations. Anidjar, in a related discussion, argues that the distinction between literal and symbolic blood is an artifact of Christianity, "an essential mechanism for the distribution and operations of blood in Christianity. . . . Blood, therefore was never a physiologic or medical substance *first*, which would *later* have acquired symbolic dimensions" (2014, 31, emphasis in original). As a metaphor, he asserts, "it does not relate to a literal term" (256). "Blood work," we could say in Latourian terms, entails both hybridization and purification. This suggests that, despite the observable processes of "purification" in the labs described in chapter 3, which aim to "objectify" blood, it can retain subject-like qualities. Blood thus repudiates the dualisms of object and subject, the material versus the immaterial.[7]

All of the qualities considered above contribute to blood's emotional salience, and evocations of blood thus have unusual political potency.[8] In a directly political context, the multitemporal evocations of blood I have described echo Katherine Verdery's discussion of the importance of temporality in a quite different bodily practice—the reburials of national figures in postsocialist Eastern Europe. Such reburials, she suggests, involve "reconfiguring time" because they both alter understandings of temporal process and involve the revision of history—and are more powerful for the fact that the revision of history had earlier been a prominent feature of Communist rhetoric and practices (1999, 112–15). Joost Fontein and John Harries (2013), following Paola Filippucci et al. (2012), suggest that it is also the openness and incompleteness of human substances, their metonymic qualities, that underlie "their resistance to processes of 'purification' and stabilization" (Filippucci et al. 2012, 211; see also Fontein and Harries 2013, 120). Bodily stuff here provides a potent set of symbolic associations that can readily link personhood, family, kinship, and nation.

Verdery's insights are taken up in Nikolai Ssorin-Chaikov's (2006) analysis of the importance of "heterochronicity" (the simultaneous coexistence of different temporal references) in Soviet displays of birthday gifts to Stalin in 1949. The rituals that Verdery and Ssorin-Chaikov examine are more organized and politically explicit reworkings of time and history than the implicit, layered invocations of blood that I discuss here. But these authors remind us of how temporality is woven into the legitimating effects of ritual (see also Bloch 1977). And Ssorin-Chaikov argues further that "heterochrony constitutes a hegemonic idiom for expressing a whole spectrum of political relationality" (2006, 371).[9] We can apply these insights to the iconic importance, mentioned above, that the blood sample of Malaysia's opposition leader, Anwar Ibrahim, suddenly assumed in the country's political crisis of 2008. According to newspaper reports, Anwar's blood (which he refused to allow the police to take) was sought, the government claimed, as an object of "scientific testing" that could be verified by "foreign experts."[10] Simultaneously, the rhetoric of politicians, as reported in the media, asserted that Anwar's blood sample had the capacity to reveal the truth about his moral status, and here the reference was apparently to a quite different and much older language and understanding of blood. But the relation between these two registers—one scientific, the other moral—and what exactly might be at stake was left almost entirely implicit in these reports. We can thus see blood as providing a particularly condensed form of the political potential of repertoires of time that are encapsulated in material objects and of the capacities of bodily matter for "meta-material" elaboration.[11] The resistance of bodily substances to any easy classification into human/ nonhuman or subject/object categories suggests that this may be a crucial aspect of their symbolic potency.

If some objects are, as Bowker and Star suggest, "naturalized in more than one world" (1999, 312), blood would seem to be a paradigmatic case of multiple naturalization. Such objects, they write, "are not then boundary objects, but rather they become standards within and across multiple worlds in which they are naturalized" (312). Their focus is on the role of boundary objects and infrastructures in classification, and they view naturalization as a key part of the process by which categories become objects that exist in different communities of practice and enable communication between them (298). This in some respects seems an apt approach to the dense flows of meaning that blood enables between different realms and its capacity for being naturalized as well as enabling further naturalizations to occur.[12] But the instability of meanings and the wide range of contexts in which blood partakes also raise questions here. The idea of a standard in a scientific sense appears to have only limited application to blood, and in highlighting temporality we have gone considerably beyond the idea of the boundary object to grasp how naturalizing processes work.

The political implications of the extraordinary metaphorical potential of blood rest partly on the conventionalization that Dedre Gentner et al. have pointed to as part of the "career of metaphor" (2001, 227). The more entangled blood's multiple resonances and metaphorical allusions become, the more familiar they seem, and the more difficult it is to see them clearly or to subject the assumptions into which they are enfolded to analytic questioning. "A naturalized object," Bowker and Star write, "has lost its anthropological strangeness. It is in that narrow sense desituated—members have forgotten the local nature of the object's meaning or the actions that go into maintaining and recreating its meaning" (1999, 299).

The work of historians in uncovering the unstable religious, familial, and political salience and embeddedness of blood in particular periods and cultural contexts in Europe is important in elucidating the force of this naturalization and its ability to enfold ideologies of exclusion (see, for example, Bynum 2007; Nirenberg 2009; Johnson et al. 2013). The reservoir of historical meanings of blood in Europe goes very deep and has retained in the twentieth and twenty-first centuries a capacity to resurface in new and powerful ways.[13] Importantly, as historians of science and medicine have shown, the scientific development of processes of transfusion, blood banking, and typing for medical purposes in the first part of the twentieth century was thoroughly culturally inflected and embedded in local histories. Such studies reveal how the trajectories of these developments were shaped by locally and historically situated understandings of, for example, "Soviet personhood" (Krementsov 2011), "race" in the US (Lederer 2008, 2013), or a supposedly egalitarian "community of strangers" in wartime Britain (Whitfield 2013). As Aihwa Ong and Nancy N. Chen (2010) show, contemporary developments of biotechnology in Asia continue to take locally specific forms and are embedded in a "situated ethics" (Ong 2010a, 12) that encompasses families, communities, and nations.

A rich body of recent anthropological literature has explored the contemporary salience of blood donation.[14] This work illuminates the myriad ways in which blood donation rests on and elaborates local practices and ideas of gift-giving, sacrifice, kinship, and ethics, as well as institutional structures, simultaneously drawing on and generating idioms and symbols with political and religious potentiality.[15] Catherine Waldby and Robert Mitchell (2006) convincingly argue that any simple dichotomous reading of blood or other tissue donation in terms of gifts versus commodities (*pace* Titmuss [1970] 1997) is inadequate to address the complexities of contemporary biotechnology practices in what they call global "tissue economies" (see also Frow 1997; Healy 2006), and to address the issues of "bioavailability" (Cohen 2005) in which tissue economies are situated. The meanings that may be ascribed to blood (or other bodily) donation, as is shown for the Malaysian case in chapter 1, exceed the conventional limits of the anthropological domains of politics, religion, economics, medical anthropology, and kinship. Conversely, rather than narrowing the range of meanings in which blood participates, medical and biotechnological practices apparently further expand its polysemous potential. But this excess also renders the symbolism of blood unstable and may have unpredictable political consequences, as was evident in the Malaysian political drama of 2008 described earlier.[16]

The development of safe procedures for the procurement and transfusion of blood in the first part of the twentieth century required its categorization into blood types and new technologies for storage (Lederer 2008, 2013; Whitfield 2013). This work of classification rested on domaining practices that would safeguard blood from contamination and minimize the occurrence of immune reactions to transfusions of the wrong type. Titmuss's contribution, referred to above, in developing policies that would best ensure the safety of donated blood by excluding payment for donation can be understood in this light. But simultaneously, as the ethnography presented in chapter 1 shows, blood donation actually requires that donors respond to familial, civic, and emotional appeals. Beyond this, it is remarkably difficult, as becomes clear in chapters 2, 3, and 4, to exclude the social world of Penang and its histories of relatedness from the spaces and work processes of the labs and blood banks. In this sense the spaces of the labs are highly ambiguous. While blood work depends on maintaining boundaries between these spaces and the outside world, the resilience of such boundaries is difficult to ensure. This is partly because medical lab technologists and other staff are social actors with their own dense networks and histories of relatedness. But it is also because the blood, which is the focus of their work, originates and is donated in social worlds.

The fact that blood is a highly visible, vital (in all senses), and naturally occurring substance heightens its capacities for symbolic elaboration (Douglas [1970] 2003) and for naturalization. What, after all, could be more obviously natural than that which is already natural? But this apparent naturalness also obscures the multiple resonances of blood. The student nurses in my opening vignette, who were nonplussed by Dr. Ho's question as to his patient's vital status, might, I suspect, have been uncertain not just about the correct answer but also about the way the question had been intended. Physical presence and symbolic potency, as we have seen, feed each other. This gives special power to metaphors of blood and enhances their potential to convey similarity and union at the same time as difference and exclusion. In an exploration of the effects of the new genetics on anglophone idioms of blood in kinship (see Finkler 2000; Rapp 1999), Sarah Franklin (2013) argues that the historical depth and embeddedness of these idioms makes them surprisingly resilient and resistant to displacement. As she trenchantly puts it, blood is "thicker than genes" (295) and for this reason, "We may be just beginning to appreciate how much more the kinship significance of blood has to teach us about understandings of genetic relations, rather than the other way around" (303).

One important feature of blood to emerge from the discussion so far is its simultaneous universality and specificity.[17] Many of its attributes, such as its plasticity, symbolic velocity, and its association with animation or its negation, can be discerned across cultures and historical eras. But the meanings and metaphors of blood are historically and culturally shaped; they have local salience and resonance and are responded to in ways that are formed in particular contexts and specific junctures. Within and beyond these spatial and temporal locations, blood both unites and divides. It can be an idiom of shared humanity or one of discrete social strata or kinds;

it can signify belonging or exclusion in terms of kinship, gender, ethnicity, "race," and nationhood. Blood is thus a powerful lens through which to examine minute social processes in what we might think of as the relatively "uncontentious spaces" of hospital clinical pathology labs or blood banks. The elusive prospect of being able to observe "naturalization in action" may be especially enticing where—as is the case for Penang—these workspaces are embedded in a social context with a long history of ethnic and religious diversity.

Penang

Penang is generally considered atypical of Malaysia. The reasons are mainly historical but have left a strong contemporary imprint. Located off the northwest coast of peninsular Malaysia in the Straits of Melaka, Penang Island (Pulau Pinang in Malay) together with its hinterland on the peninsula, Seberang Perai (formerly Province Wellesley), form the state of Penang (Negeri Pulau Pinang). Penang, Pulau Pinang, or Tanjung (in Malay, literally, "promontory," "cape," or "headland") are the terms used locally to refer to the island and to its state capital, George Town.

Formerly part of the Malay state of Kedah, Penang was established as a British colony by Francis Light in 1786. There followed an influx of migrants from other parts of the region: Kedah and other Malay states, Aceh in Sumatra, Siam, and Burma, as well as from farther afield—the Arabian peninsula, India, and China. Eurasian Catholics from Melaka, who sought refuge when the Dutch took control there from the Portuguese, were joined by Sufis from Kedah following the Siamese invasion of Kedah in 1821, which intensified migration from there (see Bonney 1971). Today the imprint of these many migratory flows can be seen in the street names and places of worship of George Town, where a dense network of streets, mosques, churches, Buddhist temples, Chinese association buildings, and Hindu temples are clustered within a short distance of each other (Tan 2009, 10–11; see also Khoo 1993).

By the early nineteenth century, the Kuan Yin temple, Kapitan Kling Mosque, Acheen Street Mosque, Nagore Shrine, Mahamariamman Temple and St. George's Church were already built at their present locations, within walking distance of one another. Nearby was the Catholic Church of the Assumption and not far away an Armenian church. Similarly assorted streams of Buddhism from Siam, Burma, Ceylon and China flowed into Penang, each with its temples and followers. (Tan 2009, 11)

Tan Liok Ee's frame of "conjunctures, confluences, contestations" illuminates how nineteenth-century flows of migration created a uniquely diverse and dynamic population in which "mixed marriages were not uncommon" (2009, 13). Arab, Indian Muslim, and some Chinese men married local women, forging economic and political bonds and giving rise to distinctive Arab and Jawi Peranakan (locally born Muslims of mixed Indian and Malay descent) and Baba-Nyonya or Peranakan (mixed Chinese Malay) populations in which different cultural elements, including cuisine, dress, and language, intermingled to create new and distinctive forms, many of which persist today (see DeBernardi 2004, 22; Tan 2009).

Demographic diversity was not, however, simply a process of blending and merging. It resulted in a plethora of different communities with their own religious, political, economic, and educational institutions. In the early twentieth century, a lively political culture and local printing presses fostered various strands of regional nationalism and modernist Islamic reform movements.[18] Religious education for rural Malays took place in Muslim *pondok* schools, Indian Muslim schools, and *madrasahs* established by Arab immigrants. Several English-language schools as well as Anglo-Chinese and Chinese schools were founded throughout the nineteenth century—many still in existence today. Schools were sites of both mixing and separation along ethnic and class lines: children of Malay, Indian Muslim, and Arab descent were brought together at Islamic institutions. Chinese schools taught children from different dialect groups and clans, while English-language education was restricted to an ethnically plural elite. Teachers came from all over the world (Tan 2009, 12–13). Apart from becoming a regional center for Islamic education, Penang was also an embarkation point and hub for pilgrims going on the Hajj from northern parts of the Malay peninsula as well as Sumatra and Siam (see Tagliacozzo 2013). In the early 1980s, villagers I knew in Langkawi who were going on the Hajj would travel first to "Tanjung."

The main impetus behind this cosmopolitan migration to Penang came from its status as a British entrepôt, the international and regional trade that passed through the island, and the economic opportunities it afforded. In 1867 Penang became a Crown colony together with Melaka and Singapore as part of the Straits Settlements. From the early nineteenth century, Singapore gradually superseded Penang as a center for international trade, but Penang remained a major hub for regional trade.[19] The cosmopolitan culture of Penang was not, however, without economic and political tensions. Concomitant with migration and urban growth, the Malay population became a minority and tended to be settled in the rural areas, while economic and cultural life in urban George Town was dominated by Arab, Jawi Peranakan, and Chinese traders with a growing body of Chinese associations (Khoo 1993). Competition over economic resources throughout the nineteenth and early twentieth centuries resulted in periodic outbreaks of violence between different secret societies involving Chinese, Malays, and Indians on both sides.[20] Religious, cultural, class, educational, and linguistic differences within what were heterogeneous Chinese, Indian, Malay, and Jawi Peranakan, or Arab, communities also mitigated against the formation of stable political alliances within and between these groups.

Occupied by the Japanese from 1941 to 1945, Penang was severely affected by World War II. The memories of this period as a time of extreme hardship are still vibrant today. When I interviewed lab staff about their family backgrounds (see chapter 2), several of them mentioned to me how their parents' education had been disrupted by the Japanese occupation. Some had family members who were part of the Communist resistance and later fought against the British in the "Malayan Emergency" of 1947–60.[21]

The political landscape of post-independence Malaysia entailed further shifts. Distinctions between "Malays," "Chinese," "Indians," and "Others," derived from colonial census categories and perceived locally in "racial" terms (see chapters 1 and 2), were inscribed in government policies, and on the identity cards required of all Malaysian citizens, as well as being constitutive of the main political parties (see Means 1976, 1991). The meanings of "race" (usually rendered as *bangsa* or *keturunan* in Malay) in successive colonial censuses, or in popular understandings in Malaysia today, have involved a complex and unstable mix of factors encompassing place of origin, descent, "nationality," culture, religion, and language, combined with the pragmatic objectives of governance.[22] The special position of Malays or Bumiputera (literally, "sons of the soil," and including some indigenous groups of Sabah and Sarawak) was enshrined in the constitution and thus rendered the position of non-Malays contingent.[23] The historical embeddedness of the "race paradigm" in Malaysia, as well as its centrality to economic policies under Prime Minister Mahathir Mohamad and his successors, and its entanglement with religion and politics, has made it particularly recalcitrant (Milner and Ting 2014; Shamsul 1998, 2001). Separation rather than confluences of political, religious, and economic life, instituted under colonial governance, has remained a dominant mode of governmentality. The history of Penang with its lively Jawi Peranakan and Straits Chinese cosmopolitan cultures (among others) is by these lights anomalous. Malay language and culture and Islam, this last seen as inseparable from Malay identity, have increasingly seemed (especially to many non-Malays) to exercise a hegemony over the existence of all Malaysian citizens.[24]

Since the 1950s, and particularly since the 1970s, the school educational system has become less diverse; teaching in public schools has occurred in the national language (Bahasa Malaysia) or, for some private schools, in English, Mandarin, or Tamil (Tan 2002; 2009, 21–22). The effects of educational policies, which favor Malay students and limit entry to universities for non-Malays,[25] impacted directly on the hospital staff whom I encountered and are discussed in chapter 2.

Penang is the only state in the Federation of Malaysia in which, historically, Malays have not constituted the majority of the population. A table in the 2010 census gave the total population of the state as 1,561,383, divided ethnically as shown in table 1.

To some extent, these distinctions map onto religious affiliations. Malays, who make up the large majority of the "Bumiputera" category, are (by definition) Muslim, while other groups have more diverse religious affiliations. The census category "Other Bumiputera" refers to non-Muslim indigenous groups that are Christian or animist. Table 4.10 of the 2010 census showed total population by ethnic group and religion for each state. In the state of Penang, most of the ethnic Chinese population was classed in the 2010 census as Buddhist (532,811 or 79.5 percent), with a minority of "Confucian, Taoist and Tribal/folk, other traditional Chinese religion" (70,237 or 10.5 percent) and Christian (59,096 or 8.8 percent). Most of the ethnic Indians were

TABLE 1. Ethnic composition of Penang, 2010

ETHNIC CATEGORY	NUMBER
Total Bumiputera	642,286
Malay	636,146
Other Bumiputera	6,140
Chinese	670,400
Indian	153,472
Others	5,365
Non-Malaysian Citizens	89,860

Source: *Population and Housing Census of Malaysia*, Department of Statistics, Malaysia 2011, 42 (table 2.10).

shown as Hindu (125,564 or 81.8 percent), with a minority of Muslims (12,335 or 8.0 percent) and Christians (10,774 or 7.0 percent) (*Population and Housing Census of Malaysia*, Department of Statistics, Malaysia 2011, 91).

Perhaps not surprisingly, given its demographic history, Penang has a tradition of political opposition to the ruling coalition that has formed the government since independence in 1957—first in the form of the Alliance comprising UMNO (the United Malays National Organisation), the MCA (Malayan Chinese Association, later Malaysian Chinese Association), and the MIC (Malayan Indian Congress, later Malaysian Indian Congress); and then, after 1969, when it was joined by Gerakan (the Malaysian People's Movement Party) and became the Barisan Nasional (National Front). From 1957 to 1966 George Town voters elected a Socialist Front coalition made up of the Labour Party and Partai Ra'ayat (later Parti Rakyat) to lead the local council. The state government of Penang was won by opposition parties in the general elections of 1969, 2008, and 2013. The results of the 2008 elections, in which the ruling Barisan Nasional lost its two-thirds majority in Parliament for the first time, constituted a major political upheaval in Malaysia and are discussed further in the section preceding chapter 3.

Economically, the development of an electronics manufacturing industry fueled growth in the 1980s and 1990s and led to the establishment and rapid expansion of new suburban areas and satellite towns and the opening of the first Penang Bridge in 1985, along with a second in 2014, linking the island by road to the mainland. The population is highly urbanized, with an urbanization rate of 90.8 percent recorded in the 2010 census (Yeoh 2014a, 249). A well-developed beach area to the northwest of the island in Batu Ferringhi, heritage sites in George Town, and the varied and high-quality cuisine for which Penang is justly famous (and in which locals take a strong interest) all contribute to the attractions that have long made the tourist industry an important part of Penang's economy. Medical tourism, although not a focus of my research, is a growing economic sector and is part of a "regional circuit" of historical connections that links Penang with Indonesia, particularly Sumatra (Whittaker, Chee, and Por 2017; see also Chee, Whittaker, and Por 2017). The island of Penang has one large public hospital, usually known as GH (General Hospital), as well as a smaller one, and at the time of my research, eight private hospitals of different sizes catering to both the local population and foreign medical tourists. Several of these were founded by religious organizations or Chinese charities.

Penang has for many decades had a lively civil society sector representing different interests, including the Consumers Association of Penang (CAP), the Penang Heritage Trust, the Women's Centre for Change, sustainable development groups, and the nonpartisan multiethnic political reform group, Aliran. Some of these groups also combine to take political initiatives under umbrella groups such as the Penang Forum. The Penang Heritage Trust was a major contributor to George Town's attainment of UNESCO World Heritage Site status together with Melaka in 2008. Unsurprisingly, rapid economic development, population growth, and transformation of the built environment have led to tensions and contestations between property development and heritage conservation (see Goh 2002; Jenkins 2008).

Penang's distinctiveness in Malaysia and the development of its trading economy, emphasized here, are clearly part of a long historical process going back to the late eighteenth century. Historians have recently begun the important work of excavating the cultural flows in different eras of the port cities of the Indian Ocean (see S. Amrith 2013; Ho 2006; Lewis 2016). Jean DeBernardi's (2004, 2006) outstanding anthropological accounts of Chinese identity formation and popular religion provide an in-depth and historically situated understanding of Chinese culture in Penang. Although the history of Penang is particular, cultural diversity is a hallmark of wider Malaysia too, especially of its urban centers, including Kuala Lumpur (see, for example, Yeoh 2014c). In the urban hinterland of Penang, on the west coast of the mainland, Donald Nonini (2015) has given a rich historical depiction of the intersection of Chinese ethnic culture and class formation, focusing on Chinese truck drivers and their bosses in the town of Bukit Mertajam. Not only do ethnicized (often racialized) identities in the form of the ubiquitous categories "Malay," "Chinese," "Indian," and "Other" thoroughly permeate many aspects of Malaysian life (see Holst 2012; chapters 1 and 2, this volume), but each category also obscures its own heterogeneous basis—as many of the aforementioned studies show. Even "Malay," a designation strongly associated with local origins, national identity, and political dominance, has been shown to rest on a history of regional demographic mobility and diversity partially obscured by strong incorporative tendencies.[26]

The complexities of cultural diversity and the separations that have been enshrined in governmentality since the colonial era have fostered an anthropology of Malaysia with a strong tendency to examine each of the main ethnic groups separately through their local, cultural, religious, or political institutions (see Yeoh 2018). My own study of Malay kinship in Langkawi (Carsten 1997) might be a case in point. This can have the effect of reproducing the already essentialized ethnic categories of government and media rhetoric as analytic frame. Nor is such ethnicization restricted to social science. Pertinently for this study, in nearby Singapore with its similar colonial and trading history, Aihwa Ong (2016, 62) has shown how an "ethnic heuristic" pervades and frames genetic research into cancer. Despite the presumed separations of ethnic difference, a corollary of the rapid urbanization, industrialization, and economic growth in Malaysia since the 1970s is that many citizens are in daily contact with "other Malaysians" of "other ethnicities" (see Kahn 2006, 154–57). This is probably especially true in contemporary urban workplaces, which are in many cases multicultural spaces. Such daily familiarity may have contributed to recent election results, which show urban voters willing to cross ethnic lines, as well as engagement in the recent movements for political reform, Reformasi, and anticorruption, Bersih. In chapter 4, I show how, although cultural practices such as postnatal prohibitions, food consumption, or ideas about ghosts are in some respects ethnically specific, they are also readily translatable between cultures. In situating much of this book in workplaces such as hospitals, blood banks, and blood donation drives, I have attempted to avoid assumptions based on an already prefigured version of what ethnicity is or how it is constituted in Malaysia. Placing ethnicity in the background, I suggest, might be a different way to reveal its contours and to see how and why it matters.

Fieldwork

The main part of the research on which this book is based took place on the island of Penang between January and July 2008; this was complemented by short visits in 2005, 2006, 2007, 2009, 2010, 2012, and 2015. The earlier visits were exploratory and were used to set up the research and find locations for fieldwork; the later ones, after I had begun writing, were to probe findings from the work carried out in 2008 and to test out initial analytical hunches. The fieldwork was based mainly but not exclusively in two medium-sized private hospitals in Penang. I have not revealed the identities of the hospitals or staff members to protect their confidentiality. While this is a necessary protocol for research, it also occludes important information. Clearly, the history of particular hospitals—their geographic location, size, the kinds of patients and population they serve in terms of class, ethnicity, and nationality, their charitable or otherwise status—matters for the processes described in this book. I did not conduct research in Penang's large public hospital, although I did visit the blood bank there. The selection of hospitals in urban Penang was partly a matter of the relative ease of acquiring research permission in different institutions, but it also resulted from my sense that, because of its size, large numbers of patients, and the pressures on staff, the public hospital would present considerable difficulties for research. The hospitals where I worked were smaller and more easy to navigate. Staff members could usually find time to talk to me. The patients who were treated in these hospitals were fairly mixed in terms of background—comprising middle- and working-class local Penangites of different ethnicities as well as some regional medical tourists, including from Indonesia and the Philippines.

Following the advice of senior doctors through whom I negotiated access, I settled initially on the clinical pathology labs as my central focus. As described in the following chapters, these labs not only ran all the diagnostic tests on blood and other bodily samples requested by doctors for hospital inpatients and outpatients; they also managed the hospital blood banks within the same spatial locations and were responsible for screening donated blood, separating it into components, and storing it. They participated in blood donation events outside the hospital, collecting blood from donors at these campaigns as well as from those who came to give blood at the hospital.

The majority of staff members of the labs were medical lab technologists, but staff also included lab technicians, phlebotomists, clerical staff, receptionists, cleaners, dispatch staff, and the lab managers. In addition, nurses, engineers, sales reps from medical technology firms, and others from inside and outside the hospital were regular visitors to these spaces. Part of the training of medical lab technologists involves periods of work placement. When groups of trainees undertook training in the labs where I was carrying out research, I discovered that their presence initiated all kinds of opportunities for discussion between them and the more senior medical lab technologists, and with myself, about the nature of their work and how it is learned, but also more generally about learning to be a responsible person and the entanglements of work, ethics, kinship, different medical systems, and other matters that this entails.

I spent much of my time in the labs, but I also accompanied lab staff or went by myself to blood donation drives located in different parts of Penang in factories, shopping malls, community halls, hospitals, and Buddhist associations. I visited hospitals and clinics outside the two hospitals that were the main focus of my research, and I spent some weeks in a dialysis center in one hospital. I accompanied medical lab technologists and phlebotomists when they went on ward rounds to collect blood samples from patients, and in general I tried to get a rounded sense of the work and lives of these enactors of "blood work" in Penang. While I was able to participate in the social life of the labs, and was remarkably free to observe the work processes that went on in these spaces and to ask questions about them, I did not directly engage in this work—so this study is based on "participant observation" of a limited kind.

The *lingua franca* of the hospitals was English, and this was the main language used in the research—though sometimes my knowledge of Malay (Bahasa Malaysia) was helpful. Beyond English and Malay, hospital staff often used other languages, especially Hokkien and Mandarin, in their communications with each other and with patients. Staff members were almost all extremely fluent in English, and many were bilingual or trilingual. The speech reproduced in the following chapters is as noted down at the time or in the following few moments. I have tried to convey the cadences, locutions, and rhythms of everyday spoken Malaysian English, which characteristically has a staccato pattern and uses direct forms and fast repartee. In this version of "Global English," pronouns, some obvious verbs, and markers of tense are often omitted. These expressive speech patterns—which might be considered a dialect or "brogue," following Marina Warner's (2016) apt usage— are markers of identity, as Warner notes, and provide a vivid entry into the worlds of experience described here.[27]

Staff members were unfailingly helpful, patient, and kind in answering my many questions and tolerating my presence. I spoke also to many blood donors in the hospitals or at other donation sites, and to patients when this did not seem to be an untoward intrusion. In addition to observing and talking about their work tasks as they were carrying them out or soon after, and engaging in informal conversations about their families and lives outside work, I conducted a set of interviews with members of lab staff to learn in more detail about their social and family backgrounds, education, and career trajectories. Toward the end of my time in Penang, I presented initial findings to lab staff and to doctors at the hospitals where I conducted the research and received extremely useful feedback.

Complementing fieldwork, I kept a file of newspaper clippings that touched on themes connected to research on blood: stories about blood or organ donation, about particular hospitals, or about medical matters more generally. As time went on, the topics of these stories became gradually more diverse as I followed the threads of conversations with blood donors, medical lab technologists, university lecturers, doctors, patients, receptionists, and the occasional proverbial taxi driver. I became aware of the ways that not only stories about blood but also wider social and political events more generally suffused these discussions and touched the lives of those to whom I spoke.

In drawing on newspaper accounts to analyze new modes of imagined criminality that emerged in Suharto's New Order Indonesia, James Siegel uses such reports to depict "the formation of a mental framework that is imposed, although in my opinion not explicitly, by one class upon another" (1998, 116). As he makes clear, the insights gained in this way emerge not by reading the newspapers alone but through his long ethnographic engagement with Indonesia. Siegel's methodological note (1998, 116–19) is pertinent. Newspaper reports are a means to access social processes not in isolation but in conjunction with the understandings gained through fieldwork (see also Gupta 1995, 377). Similarly here, such accounts are a form of public discourse that provide insights into issues, idioms, and resonances that have wide currency in Malaysia through the ethnographic work that they complement. The newspaper I have relied on most heavily is *The Star*, an English-language paper with a wide circulation in Malaysia and a historical association with Penang, from where its northern edition is published.[28] *The Star* has a broad appeal across different contexts in Malaysia; together with several Chinese-language papers, it was widely read in the hospitals and blood donation sites that I visited in Penang.

The Ebb and Flow of Chapters

The preceding discussion makes clear that this is a book about multiple interconnectedness. In the process of writing, divisions of subject matter between chapters and the directions of flow of the argument have sometimes seemed arbitrary—one might choose different beginnings or stopping points. The main ethnographic chapters focus on the details of blood donation, blood banks, and life in the clinical pathology labs. They perhaps offer a somewhat narrow ethnographic lens on Malaysia. How does this connect to dominant themes in Malaysian public life at the time of fieldwork? Each of these four ethnographic chapters is preceded by a short section drawn from newspaper accounts that explores the "public life of blood," as well as the relationship between the newspaper accounts and the enclosed world of the labs and blood banks, at the time of my research. In what ways did blood manifest itself in public discourses in Malaysia? How might such appearances resonate with work processes in the clinical pathology labs or blood banks? These sections convey the wider context of public life and events in Penang and Malaysia during the period of my research. Without affording a privileged access to the truth, newspaper accounts provide a different lens through which to calibrate the material in the ethnographic chapters.[29] They complement and broaden themes in the ethnography. What were the main issues reported in the media at this time? What were people talking about "on the street" in Penang—or at blood donation campaigns and in the blood banks and clinical pathology labs, while waiting to donate blood, during the lulls in the routine procedures of work, or over snacks, lunch, or coffee with colleagues? In describing these public events and concerns, I make connections between the seemingly rather self-contained world of the hospital labs where blood is tested, screened, and analyzed, and the wider social and political universe in which these labs exist.

Medical lab technologists, lab technicians, receptionists, lab managers, and nurses (as well as donors and patients) are directly and indirectly informed by publicity about blood donation, health scares, stories about organ donation, or hospitals that appear in the media, and by the ways these are picked up by members of the public who are also potential blood donors. And of course, as citizens, they also have multiple interests in the social and political events of Malaysian life that are carried in the local and national press. Quite by chance, as I have indicated, the period in which I conducted research in Malaysia turned out to be more politically eventful than anticipated. In the run-up to the general election of March 2008, and in the period immediately following, there was constant and lively discussion in the newspapers and more broadly about the possibility of fundamental changes to the Malaysian political scene. Wherever people met and talked, these matters were discussed with animation and interest.

At center stage were the tumultuous political events of 2008 briefly alluded to above and drawn out in the section preceding chapter 3. They included the electoral campaigns and general elections of March 2008, in which the coalition of government parties suffered a loss of electoral support but retained parliamentary power. In the aftermath, the leader of the opposition coalition, Anwar Ibrahim, was arrested and, in a bizarre reprise of events ten years earlier, during the premiership of Dr. Mahathir Mohamad, accused of sodomy (see Trowell 2015). The issue of Anwar's blood sample assumed, as we have seen, an iconic significance in these events in media reports, which also illuminates the myriad connections between blood as biomedical object and blood as a substance replete with kinship, ethnic, religious, and moral significance. In media accounts it seemed that this particular blood sample was used to question not only Anwar's moral status but also the legitimacy of political opposition to the government. But this usage appeared to have the potential to be turned back on itself and to undermine the legitimacy of the government that had set these tactics in play. The "uncontainability" of the different meanings of blood—its propensity to exceed the limits of any particular domain in which it occurs— illuminates particularly clearly the connections between such disparate fields as morality, the body, political legitimacy, and scientific testing. We can also trace such connections in the public rhetoric surrounding blood and organ donation in Malaysia. Through an examination of the terms of these morally charged discourses, we see how such topics have the potential to travel to the sites of scientific testing—into the workspaces of hospital clinical pathology labs.

In the main ethnographic chapters, my tactic has been to "follow the blood." Chapter 1 focuses on blood donors and processes of donating, and connects this to the public rhetoric surrounding blood and organ donation. The locations where blood may be donated are described, and the motivations of donors are depicted through different donor stories. Here ideas about health, kinship ties, and memories of kinship are revealed as salient. The donor booklet has particular significance as an artifact that encapsulates a donor's life story. Acts of blood donation involve categorization, and the forms completed by donors constitute another kind of crucial artifact that permits further acts of classification. The donor form classifies donors according to age, gender, and ethnicity, but the relation between what is stated on the form and the donor thus categorized is not always straightforward. The forms record donors as "voluntary," "replacement," or "autologous" and as "regular" or "first-time." These classifications are important to the pathways on which blood travels in the lab. The distinction between voluntary and replacement donors reveals a tension surrounding the nonmonetary payment and gifts that voluntary donors receive in return for their blood. The problematic status of blood and its capacity to reveal or generate moral properties is further illuminated by the difficulties that ensue when some donors are rejected by blood bank staff as unsuitable for donation.

Chapter 2 introduces the workspaces and the staff of the labs and blood banks. The spaces are depicted in terms of the apparently clear boundaries that demarcate them within the hospitals and in terms of the divisions of space that underlie work processes. But we also begin to discern the ambiguities of these spaces, where boundaries are at best provisional, and which are at once alien and unfamiliar but carry traces of domesticity. The discussion then focuses on medical lab technologists and the particular niche they occupy in terms of educational backgrounds, training, and work. Staff members' age, gender, education, class, and ethnicity, with its strong religious associations, are set against broader features of contemporary urban Malaysia and examined in terms of how they reflect social mobility over the last few decades. Different personality types that are particularly drawn to laboratory work are discussed. But the usefulness of such typologies can also be queried—and this is partly because of the apparently contradictory demands of this work, which encompass both technical tasks and sociability, aspects pursued further in chapters 3 and 4.

What happens to blood when it enters the lab and blood bank? The analysis in chapter 3 shifts to the work that goes on in the labs and to processes of categorization and diagnosis. I describe how "objective" blood and blood products are created through the screening and testing of blood and its separation into blood products. The label is introduced as a crucial artifact that ensures the safety and reliability of processes of testing, screening, and cross-matching. The objective appearance of the sample in its labeled test tube may, however, be undermined by resonances of social relations that travel between lab staff and the products they analyze. Here I draw on Annemarie Mol's (1998, 2002) discussion of "multiple" and "unstable" objects to probe the nature of the sample and the way ethics and politics are enfolded into laboratory work. One important facet of medical lab technologists' work is the collection of blood from donors, outpatients, and patients in the hospital wards. This initiates a space for interaction between donors and those who collect blood. How this space is traversed and the kinds of interaction that ensue suggest further ambiguities and tensions over what is involved in these exchanges. Issues of contamination and contagion and the risks and dangers of the workplace are discussed. I use the notion of "rehumanization" to depict some of the ways in which social expectations and obligations seep into laboratory life. This includes how medical lab technologists actively track individual cases or samples that arouse their interest or that derive from people they know or to whom they are related, and in so doing may improve the quality of work. Patients may sometimes be colleagues and also relatives, and this crucially affects the nature of the workplace. Further, learning and training in the lab are revealed to be highly social rather than merely technocratic endeavors. The discussion illuminates the seepages and pathways for different kinds of social knowledge to travel with samples or donated blood as they make their way around the lab.

Chapter 4 depicts the sociality of the labs through the lives and relationships of those who work there. As one medical lab technologist put it to me, "Work is just a small part of the job," and in this chapter we encounter some surprising and unorthodox presences in laboratory life. Eating, which is not permitted in the working spaces, is one paradoxical focus of the sociality of the labs. Kinship and marriage have an equally surprising presence and can be understood in part as a temporal extension of the commensal relations of work. The notion of "domestication" captures the way these processes mitigate the alien and risky aspects of work and the spatial ambiguities of the clinical pathology labs. Ideas about health and illness, including postnatal confinement and prohibitions, in which blood is crucial, reveal some unexpected dissonances between different kinds of knowledge available to medical lab technologists. Lab staff often treat themselves using traditional Chinese, Ayurvedic, and other non-Western kinds of medicine. Religious experience and ethical engagement are also important dimensions of medical lab technologists' lives and are described through lab workers' obligations and commitments outside the hospital. Finally, we turn to the disputed and much-discussed presence of ghosts in the lab and to the question of what this reveals about the risks and dangers of these workspaces and their fragile boundaries.

In the conclusion, I return to the general and particular salience of this study, drawing together the various themes of the chapters to show how efforts to separate "socially embedded" from "objective" blood are both intrinsic to the work of the lab and also inherently unstable, constantly threatening to unravel. This is partly because they are enacted by social actors who are embedded in multiple locations and relations within and outside the lab. It is also because the collection of blood in fact relies on the effectiveness of rhetoric about ethical sharing and helping others, or saving a life, through which blood donation is encouraged (as described in chapter 1). And these interconnections are further amplified through the wider political salience of such rhetoric. Blood's participation in many domains and its importance as a medium of communication between them mean that boundaries are difficult to maintain—as the disputed presence of ghosts in the lab eloquently signifies. At the same time, routine checks and controls over work tasks limit the porosity of such boundaries and the potentially devastating consequences of compromising the safety of blood products and of lab and blood bank procedures.

Finally, the discussion returns to the wider issues raised in this introduction about the nature of blood. Many of the ethnographic details presented in this study are specific to Malaysian sociality or political life, but their significance is broader. Neither the aptitude of blood for metaphoric extension nor the importance of safeguarding blood products and ensuring the accuracy of testing and diagnosis are restricted to the Malaysian context. The patient in the operating room on a heart-lung machine, depicted at the start of this chapter, whose blood has been moved beyond the body is, as Dr. Ho noted, "in limbo"—neither alive nor dead. The exceptional properties of blood, including its animating potential and its tendency to flow between domains and temporalities, accruing, sedimenting, and transferring resonances, have implications both for its symbolic power and for its status as a biomedical object. Blood's unusual propensity to be "naturalized in more than one world," one starting point for this intellectual journey, means that it may, literally, be uncontainable.

● ● ●

In their introduction to a collection of critical essays on the place of kinship in modernity, Susan McKinnon and Fenella Cannell (2013) argue that the separation between kinship and other aspects of social life—economics, politics, the realm of science, the workplace—should be understood as part of the ideology of modernity rather than its lived reality. They are critical of the "crypto-progressivism" of Michel Foucault ([1978] 1979, 1985, 1991) and scholars influenced by him whose focus on regimens of governmentality assumes that kinship has been displaced from institutions of liberal modernity by "biopower" and "biological citizenship" (McKinnon and Cannell 2013, 35).[30] Their nuanced discussion builds on earlier feminist scholarship on processes of naturalization in gender and kinship and on the assumptions and effects of the separation of anthropological subject matter into distinct analytic domains, such as gender, kinship, politics, and economics (see Yanagisako and Delaney 1995).

McKinnon and Cannell suggest that a long-overdue project is to subject the role of kinship *within* self-consciously modern institutions and processes to proper scrutiny. In their edited collection, twenty-first-century transnational silk firms in Italy and China (Yanagisako 2013), outsourced shipyards in India (Bear 2013), and Argentinean petroleum production (Shever 2013) are revealed to have kinship enfolded within the very core of the productive relations of contemporary capitalism, but these are often heavily obscured and mainly hidden from view. In the more historical essays in their volume, however, we can discern the processes through which kinship and the political economy are teased apart—for example, in the anxieties surrounding the growth of Mormonism in late nineteenth-century North America (Cannell 2013).

In a poignant case central to the origins of kinship studies in anthropology, Gillian Feeley-Harnik (2013) excavates the Lewis Henry Morgan papers at the University of Rochester, in upstate New York, to show how Morgan's own research trajectory was intimately entangled with his family life. She reveals that the dedication that Morgan originally wrote for *Systems of Consanguinity and Affinity of the Human Family* (Morgan 1871) to his two young daughters—who had died within a month of each other from scarlet fever in 1862 while Morgan was on a field trip to the American West—was removed by Joseph Henry, secretary of the Smithsonian Institution, as "unscientific." Morgan had described *Systems* as "equally their contribution . . . to the Science of the Families of Mankind" (Morgan Papers Box 12:2, p. 7, cited in Feeley-Harnik 2013, 180). Feeley-Harnik notes, "Lewis saved the drafts of his dedication and his sketches for the crypt and his daughter's sarcophagi [at Rochester's Mount Hope cemetery] with his manuscript of *Systems* and other papers, and he willed them with money for the education of women to the University of Rochester, where they can still be found" (2013, 180).

The anxiety to separate Morgan's "scientific" work from his personal connections, Feeley-Harnik argues, came at a particular historical juncture. It was one expression of a larger, self-consciously modernizing endeavor to separate different kinds of humanity, and newly emerging forms of labor and property arrangements, including slavery and its abolition. New forms of personhood went hand in hand with the spatial reorganization of northeastern American cities, including Rochester, into separate residential and business districts with new parks and cemeteries. These "moral-political-economic processes," she suggests, were part of the "inseparable" development of kinship and capitalism in late nineteenth-century America (Feeley-Harnik 2013, 212). Feeley-Harnik's attentiveness to such myriad and simultaneous spatial, economic, intellectual, familial, and emotional fault lines alerts us to how these are together the outcome of underlying historical developments.

The work of "domaining," which is part of the performance and ideology of modernity (McKinnon and Cannell 2013; Yanagisako and Delaney 1995), runs counter to an ongoing process of connection that constitutes sociality, and which occurs in idioms of commensality, kinship, religion, ethnicity, or nationhood—or a mixture of any of these. Blood is one medium of connection that places these supposedly separate domains in mutual communication. And this is why observing blood work in Penang—where, side by side and in constant traffic with each other, we find idioms of science and family, truth and food, professional life and everyday joking—offers possibilities for elucidating domaining and naturalization in a new light.

But beyond this, the ethnography in this book shows what the highly routinized, impersonal, and often uninspiring work of the labs and the medical demand for donated blood require to be well performed. The tasks of donation, sample collection, testing, monitoring, screening, labeling, and cross-matching, in their minute exactitude, rely on the active and continued engagement of those who perform them. Purification, in the Latourian sense, does not in any straightforward way ensure the quality of blood work. It is in the moments of slippage when we perceive echoes of ghosts, food, kinship, memory, and care in the labs that this becomes most clear. Rather than being purified out, the apparently inimical elements of blood work— the banter, food, religion, discussions of marriage, race, lotteries, scandals, and ghosts—turn out to be part of the vital lifeblood of these ultramodern spaces and paragons of modernity, the hospital clinical pathology labs.

Blood in this book thus stands for the messy, sticky, and binding social glue that is necessary to make modern institutions such as hospitals, blood donation centers, labs, or science work well. It both elucidates the myth of domaining under modernity and shows its tangential relevance to the version that is Malaysia's particular modernization project.[31] The multifaceted and plural meanings of blood indeed encapsulate the "mystery," alluded to by Kuriyama (2002) and captured in the vignette at the beginning of this introduction, of what separates the living and the dead. This is what is expressed when lab staff articulate its ambiguously animated status and its unique truth-bearing qualities. Social scientists too, I suggest, can learn from blood's capacity to reveal interconnections between actors, sites, terrains of knowledge, and discourses that sometimes give the illusory appearance of being strictly separated.

On April 2, 2008, an article headed "Donating Blood for 26 Years" in *The Star* described how "traffic police officer L/Kpl Nekmat Monil has been donating blood for 26 years and he was not going to let a broken arm stop him."

> "After learning about the blood donation drive, I could not wait to do the needful," he said, adding that the only time he skipped an occasion to donate blood was when he was injured in an accident in 2005.
>
> The father of four said he felt it was his duty to donate blood.
>
> "I believe that I can help a lot of people. As long as I can help others, I don't mind doing it," he said.[1]

The report described how this blood donation drive had been organized "in conjunction with the 201st Police Day celebration," at which "100 police officers" had donated blood. A police superintendent underlined how "the campaign was one of the activities held to foster ties between the public and the police force."[2] A similar event at which 300 donors gave blood, including "Butterworth Court prosecuting officer, Chief Insp N Govindarajan, 38, and his wife, R. Mathurakala, 36[,] a teacher," was covered in May. The chief inspector, "a regular donor," was reported as saying, "I hope more policemen will come forward to donate for a good cause."[3]

Visiting Malaysia shortly before Ramadan in 2007, I was struck by the almost daily reports on blood drives in the newspapers and the accompanying exhortations to donate. Blood donation campaigns are often advertised in advance in the local sections of newspapers. Such notices intensify just before and during Ramadan, when a fall in donations from Malays results in severe shortages. At all times of the year, successful and more high-profile blood donation campaigns appear in the newspapers with brief stories and photos highlighting the number of donors who have come to give blood.

I was intrigued by what particularly Malaysian resonances such reports might convey.

In themes replicating those that came to the fore in conversations with donors and blood bank staff, as described in chapter 1, these reports highlighted the number of donors at campaigns, as well as the idea that some were "regular donors" who had an extraordinary history of donation—they had given blood many times, over many years. Other newspaper reports on blood donation campaigns included one jointly organized by the Penang branch of a national bank and an automobile company at which "free souvenirs such as towels, umbrellas, and coin boxes were given to donors." "Among the donors" at this event "was EON Penang branch sales manager Nazrim Bin Mohamad Yusoff. It was his third time after he had donated twice for his parents."[4] Articles such as these touched on the ways that blood donation could be embedded in kinship relations and on the rewards donors received. Another report on June 28 mentioned that "the Taiping Lake Hash House Harriers and Harriets Club recently organised a blood donation drive in conjunction with Mother's Day and Father's Day."[5] Describing how more donors than anticipated had come to this event, "Club joint master N. Morgan" was reported as saying, "now we have 68 donors as some of our members brought along their friends, relatives or neighbours."[6]

Some reports seemed to imply that the resonances of blood donation might stretch beyond "helping others" and connotations of kinship and other ties of sociality that were regularly mentioned. An article in *The Star* on June 2, 2008, was headed "Members Who Have Paid Can Vote Elsewhere." The accompanying photograph showed a blood donor giving blood surrounded by a doctor and various dignitaries. The caption under the photo read, "Good response: Lam Wah Ee consultant pathologist Prashanta K. Das (left) checking a blood donor. Also present are Koay (second right) and Lions Club of Penang Gold Coast chapter president Francis Goh (third left)." Significantly, however, the focus of the article was a political discussion with a local Penang MCA (Malaysian Chinese Association) official. The MCA, part of the government alliance, Barisan Nasional, had suffered severe losses at the general elections in March. The article began, "MCA life members and those who have paid their annual subscription fees can vote at other branches if their own branch has been disqualified from holding the party election after failing to collect the minimum annual subscription to operate."

It went on to describe how "Penang MCA Bukit Gelugor division chairman Datuk Koay Kar Huah" had talked to reporters after launching a blood campaign at Lam Wah Ee Hospital. Barely mentioning the blood campaign, the article concluded, "Koay had not given up his hope on the party after their severe defeat in the general election but would continue to contribute to the party and would fight to wrestle back the seats that they had lost."[7] It was perhaps partly the fact that blood donation campaigns were public events, which sometimes featured local dignitaries and might be the occasion for speeches, that made it easy to connect blood donation to such overtly political matters.

But there were further matters at stake. During an exploratory visit to Penang in 2005, I had found the medical practitioners to whom I talked interested in my proposed research because, in their view, the local shortage of donated blood was a result of "cultural factors" inhibiting willingness to donate blood or to receive it from particular sources. This suggested some specifically Malaysian issues surrounded donation, and newspaper reports corroborated this. That ethnicity is highlighted in bodily exchanges was reflected in local media coverage of a heart transplant operation that took place in Kuala Lumpur in October 2007. Newspaper reports highlighted the fact that one of the two donors was Malay, while the teenage girl who was the recipient was Malaysian Chinese. Nor was the opportunity for making political mileage out of this missed by leaders, who praised such testimony to harmonious interethnic relations. Thus one newspaper article headed "Transplant Touches Hearts," reported,

> Umno Youth chief Datuk Seri Hishammuddin Tun Hussein said the noble deed of a Malay boy's family donating his heart to Hui Yi transcended race and religion. "It is so special and touching. In a time when there are issues relating to racial and religious divisions. The act has given us hope. This is exactly what the Barisan Nasional [National Front] tries to do. We need to highlight more such stories," said Hishammuddin at the opening of the Gerakan Youth and Wanita delegates' conference at Menara PGRM yesterday.

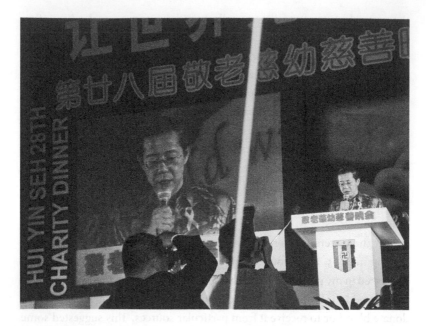

The Chief Minister of Penang gives a speech at a charity dinner for blood donors.

The same article began,

> The double transplant case of 14-year old Tee Hui Yi had the Gerakan
> Youth delegates and VIPs engrossed yesterday. Tan Sri Dr Koh Tsu Koon
> said a heart transplant was more dramatic than blood donation, which
> was now a normal procedure. "When blood is transfused into one's body,
> no one would ask whether this is blood from a Chinese or Malay. To
> all of us, it is just human blood," he said, adding that Malaysians should
> be grateful for the advances. "There are many things we have taken for
> granted. Mutual help and inter-marriages, it is happening in this coun-
> try," he said.[8]

In these politically inflected commentaries, the connections between
organ transfers, blood donation, and harmonious ethnic relations, encompassing cooperation and intermarriage, are laid out in a logically implied
sequence that is also a moral discourse.

Tee Hui Yi's progress continued to be reported in the press in 2008. An
article headed "Happy to Be Home Again," described how she was cele-

brating Chinese New Year at home with her family. Her mother, the article stated, "said it was a dream come true to have her daughter home with her to celebrate Chinese New Year with the entire family."

> She also expressed her heartfelt gratitude to all Malaysians who supported Hui Yi and the entire family through her daughter's illness.
>
> "Everyone, irrespective of race, prayed for Hui Yi. Thank you so much," she said, adding that she was so grateful to MCA President Datuk Seri Ong Ka Ting who had assured her that he would help her family out in every way.[9]

Just a few days before the general election on March 8, a further report, titled "A 'New' Birthday for Hui Yi," described how her father, Tee Ah Soon, had decided that Hui Yi's birthday would thenceforth be celebrated on October 5, the day of her second heart transplant operation, to mark her "rebirth," instead of on March 14, her actual birthday. Curiously enough, the central message seemed once again to be a political one:

> Tee thanked the Barisan Nasional government, especially MCA president Datuk Seri Ong Ka Ting and former Health Minister Datuk Seri Dr Chua Soi Lek for the help and support in Hui Yee's [sic] recovery.
>
> Tee has also pledged his vote for incumbent Parit Yaani state assemblyman Ng See Tiong when the latter visited the family in Parit Besar here yesterday.[10]

And the accompanying photograph showed the state assemblyman presenting a bouquet of flowers to Hui Yi while her parents and others looked on.

While this report was carried in the national news section, on the same day, the local news section of *The Star* carried another article headlined "Paying Tribute to Muslim Couple," with a line underneath, "Donating son's heart transcends race and religion, says Ka Chuan." The report began,

> The selfless act of a Muslim couple who donated their brain dead son's heart to save Tee Hui Yi's life has touched many people and it has reflected the spirit of Malaysia—a good deed which transcends race and religion.

"We need more of such warm and selfless acts to develop Malaysia," said Datuk Ong Ka Chuan, Barisan Nasional candidate for Tanjung Malim parliamentary seat.

"Let us all work together to bring harmony and development of the country to greater heights," he said.[11]

These excerpts make clear the capacity of blood and organ donation to function as a symbolic vector that moves with apparent ease between issues of health, matters of life and death (encompassing "rebirth"), the family, selfless giving, and a "spirit of Malaysia." It is no accident that the spirit of Malaysia embodied by such a "warm and selfless act," and alluded to three days before the general election, should above all have been one that "transcends race and religion," the implied sources of disharmony. And what could be more apt as a symbol of such transcendence than a heart donated across the lines of religion and ethnicity? It is a short leap to suggest that such rebirth, and future "harmony and development," are bound up in a vote for the governing Barisan Nasional. The repeated allusions to racial and religious divisions by politicians imply of course a threat of the chaos and disorder that may ensue if the government should lose. While the rhetoric apparently states that Malaysian citizens can and should rise above such differences, it simultaneously rests on an essentialist vision of the world in which these distinctions are ever-present and might potentially engulf the nation, especially if votes are cast for the wrong parties.

The language in these accounts is perhaps familiar. What is striking is the ease with which a space for blood or organ donation can be made within it. While the politicians made much of the Malay Muslim donor's family and their gift across "racial" and religious lines, that of the second donor (required because the first heart was rejected) was barely mentioned in these reports and was not the subject of political speeches. It seems that blood and organs have an unusual symbolic weight and that their connotations are particularly amenable to creative adaptations.

There was steady coverage in the Malaysian press in 2008 of the shortage of organ donors both in Malaysia and abroad. The *New Straits Times* reported that the Singapore government's Human Organ Transplant Act, which for the previous twenty years had meant that those between the ages of twenty-one and sixty were presumed to have agreed to the donation of vital organs upon death unless they had opted out, was extended on August 1, 2008, to include Muslims. This involved local Islamic authorities in Singapore issuing an edict to allow Muslims to be included.[12] Discussions about possible incentives to increase the pool of donors in Malaysia and more widely were reported regularly, with special reference to high numbers of patients in Malaysia on dialysis who might be suitable for kidney transplants. Newspaper reports also paid attention to "barriers" to donation, including "cultural" factors, such as religion, as well as legislative and infrastructural ones.[13]

Other articles gave publicity to the families of donors and the value of donating[14] or reported in negative terms on the families of would-be donors who had failed to honor their pledges. A report headed "Dismal Donor Numbers," with the subheading "Parents Refuse to Honour Children's Pledge after Deaths," in *The Star* on May 15, 2008, recorded,

> Penang Hospital Nephrology Services head Datuk Dr Rozina Ghazalli said according to Health Ministry records, 112,300 Malaysians had pledged to donate their organs from 1997 till March 31 this year.
>
> "However, the actual donors was only 214 from 1976 till March 31 this year," she told *The Star* in an interview here on Tuesday.

Reporting the reasons for the reluctance of family members "to allow doctors to remove the organs of their beloved ones," and also the failure of doctors to explain properly the meaning of brain death, the article continued,

> "In such instances, the doctors do not want to be seen as vultures waiting to get the deceased person's organs or to be seen as not doing their best to save the patient's life," she said.
>
> And commenting on the low numbers of Muslim donors,
>
> Dr Rozina said although all religions encourage the act of compassion to save lives, Muslims in particular were still reluctant to donate organs.
>
> "They think it is disrespectful for the dead to be buried with organs missing although there is a *fatwa* which allows Muslims to donate their organs," she said.

According to the statistics cited in this report, the number of pledges by Muslims had increased from 2 percent in 1997 to 12 percent in 2007. "The highest number of actual donors were Chinese (52.4%) followed by Indians (26.6%) and Muslims (6.1%)."[15] This article vividly substantiates a recognizably Malaysian set of associations. As a straightforward, factual account of the shortage of donors in Malaysia, it apparently aimed to encourage potential donors from all backgrounds to come forward—the report concluded with hospital contact details, including phone numbers, for "those interested in becoming a donor." In discussing the possible reasons for a shortage of donors, cultural factors come into play, including the reasons for relatives refusing consent even when organs have been pledged. From the wishes of family members it seems an obvious step to turn to religious matters. And thus the discussion moves to Muslim donation and then to statistics that apparently conflate ethnic and religious identity, giving figures for "Chinese," "Indians," and "Muslims." We will see that this is a habitual way of presenting matters in Malaysia. Indeed, these very connections, encompassing family, religion, ethnicity, and "race," are relied on in the political commentaries referred to above. The same set of conventional associations is evident at many points in the following chapters. Thus in chapter 1 we see its prominence in the way acts of donation are recorded on blood donation forms, and also in the capacity of large-scale blood donation events to absorb or promulgate political messages; chapter 2 depicts its importance for staff in the labs and blood banks; chapter 3 shows how these associations permeate the intricate work processes of the labs; and in chapter 4 we see how it is refracted in processes of sociality among lab staff.

ONE

Blood Donation

A Tale of Two Donors

One morning in March 2009, a man in his mid-fifties arrived at one of the blood banks that I was observing to give blood, as he explained proudly, for the 104th time in his life. Dressed in shorts, a polo shirt, and flip-flops, he began a voluble and lively monologue on his history of donating blood. The donor booklets he carried, clipped together, attested to a long history of donating blood stretching back thirty-two years, which encompassed not just several hospitals in Penang but also others in different states of peninsular Malaysia. Along with his donor booklets, he carried other mementoes of his previous donations: certificates from hospitals, bus tickets to neighboring states, photographs of one of the hospitals that he favored, an envelope that had held a supermarket voucher given as a token of appreciation by one of the blood banks, a special cup that was a souvenir for regular donors from another hospital. He carefully unwrapped these various artifacts from document cases, envelopes, and boxes and displayed them in response to my interest, while lamenting the loss of an inscribed donor's T-shirt, a reward from one blood bank that, he said, had been stolen by a drug addict. I was struck not just by the expansive detail in which this man told me about his history of blood donation but also by how truncated his answers became when I asked him about his family. His wife had died twenty-five years before, he told me, and his only daughter did not live with him. Whereas for many donors it seemed easy to locate their acts of donations in stories of kinship and family lives, which were part of their personal significance, for this person, it seemed as though the value of blood donation had expanded to become the guiding principle that gave meaning to his life.

The embeddedness of acts of donation in particular lives, histories of kinship, and moral discourses was made more complex by the fact that the hospitals where I was located not only took blood from voluntary donors but also operated a system of requesting replacement donations from the families of patients who needed blood transfusions. Some donors had therefore been strongly encouraged to donate by staff keen to maintain the supply of blood available in the hospital blood banks. At the same time that the enthusiastic voluntary donor whom I have just described was expanding on his life history of donation, on the bed next to him in the blood bank another person was also donating blood. In marked contrast to his neighbor, this was a young man who spoke very little and who was clearly feeling quite unwell after donating. Several times, he tried to get up from the bed where he was resting but was seemingly overcome by nausea and giddiness. His mother, who accompanied him, explained that her son was there as a replacement donor for his grandmother, a patient at the hospital, and that he had a phobia about giving blood. On learning that this young man was giving blood for the first time and was clearly suffering the consequences, his older, more voluble, and more experienced neighbor on the next bed told him that if he gave blood more often he would become accustomed to it, and it would get easier. He too had been very tired the first time he had given blood, he said, but in time his body had adjusted to donating every three months. In fact, giving blood was a bit like tapping rubber from a rubber tree—it would quickly be replenished.

These two contrasting cases highlight just some of the differences between donors, as well as the fact that replacement donors may be subject to persuasion from family or friends. But as commentators pointed out to me, the contrast could also be misleading since voluntary donors are also subject to constraints or persuasion of various kinds. Notoriously, the army and police in Malaysia are on occasion more or less ordered to give blood—on a "voluntary" basis. And one university lecturer recalled that when she had been up for promotion and had nothing much to write under the heading "community service," she had been advised that the easiest thing to do would be to donate blood at the university clinic. So between "saving a life," "doing good," "helping others," and other such statements of virtuous altruism, and acting as a replacement donor (or donating more or less on order), a variety of motivating factors come into play. These might include the material signs of recognition with which blood banks sometimes reward donors, such as certificates, special T-shirts, and the like, as well as more overtly financial recompense, including supermarket vouchers, or outwardly less visible monetary compensation from the families of patients receiving blood transfusions. While for many donors less tangible emotions of pride or satisfaction are the central consequences of donating, other factors clearly also play their part. And in many cases, as I will elaborate, these complex motivations are also woven into career paths and family histories.

• • •

This chapter examines the social life of blood from the point of view of donors and of the staff who take their blood. As the above vignette makes clear, the process of donation is an ambivalent one, capable of being read in multiple ways. In order to tease apart these nuances, I begin by describing some of the locations where blood donation takes place and the different contexts in which it occurs. I then examine some of the ways blood donors are categorized and the motivations they articulate for giving blood. What kinds of stories lie behind a willingness to donate blood? The different types of motivation at play—from the altruistic to the more self-interested—feed into a tension between payments and gifts that underlies the practices and discourses surrounding blood donation. Here social exchanges that are endowed with a positive moral aura through the rhetoric of gift-giving or saving a life can be shown to entail more ambiguous and morally loaded judgments and expectations. While Richard Titmuss's ([1970] 1997) pathbreaking study emphasized the morality of the "gift relationship" as ensuring the safety of donated blood and its products, we see how the blood donation is a far from simple act and that an adequate understanding of it entails looking beyond the rhetoric of the gift to "the fine texture of life" (Das 2000, 284; see also Waldby and Mitchell 2006). The gift of blood donation is socially embedded in myriad ways and has the capacity to carry with it some of the personal qualities and history of the donor—in other words, to be gift-like in a more Maussian sense than Titmuss's utopian vision intended.[1]

Preceding donation, a form must be completed by all intending donors and is handed in to blood bank staff. But the relations among the information on the form, the donor, and blood that is given are by no means transparent. Taking the form as a kind of "boundary object" (Bowker and Star

1999), which should standardize and also stabilize the meanings of blood embedded in donation, I look at the kinds of information that the form requires intending donors to supply, the possible answers that may be given, and what happens to this information once the form is completed. Donors themselves can be categorized in various different ways—and the donor form is one means by which such categorizations occur. Potential blood donors are assessed and sometimes turned away by blood bank staff. Some donors have long-term knowledge of those who work in the blood bank, and this can create complex scenarios if staff members feel they should refuse a donor. Such refusals are not always easy for staff to negotiate and must be seen as part of the nexus of social exchanges in which blood is situated. Once it has been donated, blood itself is labeled by blood group, screened, and separated into blood products. But other processes of categorization precede, accompany, and underlie the division of blood into particular categories. Different kinds of hospitals, contexts and modes of donation, as well as different sorts of donors and types of recompense are, as I will show, interwoven in histories of blood-taking.

Alongside the categorization of blood into blood groups, its screening and separation into blood products is a nuanced process of social engagement and distinction that I trace here. Blood itself is multiply embedded in layers of social processes and relationships. The rhetoric of gift-giving and saving a life thus overlays a range of scenarios and exchanges encompassing more coercive or nonvoluntary giving, different forms of nonmonetary recompense, and the difficulty of refusing donors. The transfer of blood to the blood bank and clinical pathology labs involves, by contrast, an attempt to sever these links and obliterate the social traces of donated blood (see chapter 3). Partly because of the imperative to safeguard patients from contamination, and because of the involvement of staff who are themselves social actors, this process of "recategorizing" blood, or re-creating it as an "objective" medical entity, following donation is by no means absolute or complete. The resonances and qualities which blood carries are, it would seem, too powerful to be effectively dispelled through the use of boundary objects and infrastructures. Its social embeddedness occurs in too many domains, and is too multilayered, to be easily disentangled or erased. Blood, as we shall see, has a tendency to overflow its boundaries.

Locations

There are many ways to give blood in Malaysia. These range from the most impromptu private gesture executed by lone individuals, simply by going to a hospital blood bank as in my opening vignette, to more populous "spectacles" of blood donation performed in various kinds of public places (including shopping malls, community halls, and temples) and involving several hundred people over the course of a half day or longer. I observed a variety of these sites during my fieldwork in Penang but by no means exhausted the possibilities available to donors. In the hospitals where I was based, intending donors could also come to the blood bank at any time during working hours to donate blood. Blood banks had a slow trickle of intending donors (generally just a few people on most days) who came to donate blood either alone, or sometimes with a spouse, or as a group of friends or colleagues. These donors included members of the public with no particular connection to the hospital, friends or relatives of hospital inpatients who had been encouraged to donate blood, and hospital staff, especially student nurses from the hospital nursing colleges, who were also encouraged to give blood.

The hospitals to which I was attached were small to medium-sized private institutions. Their blood banks had just a few beds to accommodate donors, and they usually had just one or two people on duty in the blood bank. Large-scale blood donation campaigns were organized in various ways. On some occasions a mobile blood campaign was set up by the hospital at a particular factory or other place of work. Workers were offered various kinds of health checks in return for donating blood, for example, blood pressure and blood sugar level checks or breast screening. Some of these were given free, others were paid for at a reduced rate. Workers might also be given a talk on some aspect of health care by one of the hospital doctors.

Other kinds of blood donation campaigns were organized by various civic organizations, such as the Lions Club, Buddhist charitable associations, and associations whose function was to encourage blood donation, with the participation of local hospitals. These were held at different venues, including hospitals, association premises, or community halls. Larger-scale events involved the collaboration of two or three hospitals and were held in large halls. The staff from the blood banks of two or three different hospitals

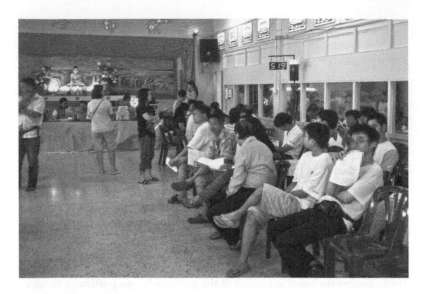

Donors wait to give blood at a mass blood drive.

would set up separate long tables for processing intending donors on opposite sides of the hall. Donors would first fill in their donor forms; they would have a short conversation about their answers either while filling in the form or immediately afterward, usually with one of the personnel from the voluntary organization involved, or sometimes with one of the hospital staff. These conversations were not necessarily completely private, as there were often people milling around or the donor was accompanied by members of his or her family.

Having filled in the form, donors would wait in rows of seats before being called forward for their predonation checks. These were carried out by lab staff and nursing students. Intending donors would proceed along one side of a row of tables, where staff members were seated in pairs on the other side carrying out the necessary checks. First, blood pressure was taken and noted by one pair, then hemoglobin level, and then the donor's blood group was ascertained. Once all the checks had been carried out, the donors would proceed with their form to the blood donation area. Here rows of folding beds would be set up—the different hospitals would each occupy different areas of one hall. Waiting donors would sit on seats near

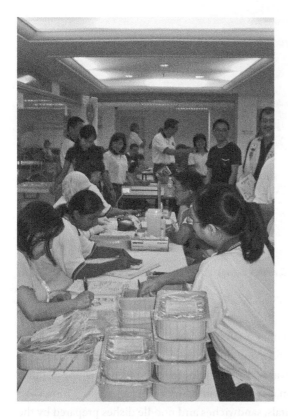

Donors queue for pre-donation tests.

each hospital's beds and would be called forward when the staff from the hospital blood bank and clinical pathology labs were ready. Because of the numbers of people being processed, donors sometimes spent several hours at these events. Once a bed became available, the donor would lie down; the lab staff would swab their arm, anesthetize it, and insert a needle attached to a tube and blood bag. Donors were usually then given a small box or bag with various small gifts or a drink and a sandwich in it.

At many of the blood campaigns I attended, cooked food was served to donors and those accompanying them in a separate area. At the blood campaigns held at the hall of one Buddhist association, women from the association cooked various noodle dishes in large pans in the kitchen at the back, and food and cold drinks were served to donors and their families in a room off the main hall in a quite informal way, with some people sitting

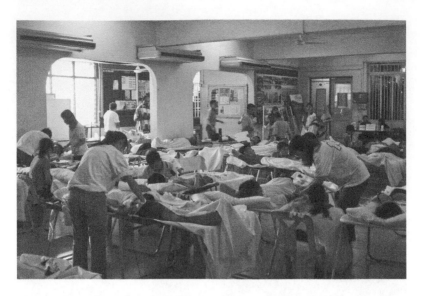

Mass blood donation event with donors on beds.

and some standing in a rather small space. At a blood campaign to honor donors who had given blood many times, which I attended on the mainland, a more elaborate meal was set out at tables for donors and visiting political dignitaries. And at a smaller-scale donation organized by the Lions Club within one of the hospitals, sandwiches and noodle dishes prepared by the hospital canteen as well as warm and cold drinks were served. Some but not all of these events also included speeches.

I take up in more detail below some aspects of the blood donation events that I have described, including the various kinds of exchanges within which they are embedded and the classification of donors through the information they write on their forms. Here I emphasize their flexibility of scale and content: they may constitute private and solitary acts undertaken by an individual at a convenient moment by quietly visiting their local hospital on the way to or from work or on a day off. But they may also involve hundreds of people and combine aspects of political events or civic or social gatherings harnessed to particular causes. Donation events are particularly appropriate for such enlargement because the rhetoric surrounding blood and organ donation is always already phrased in terms of saving a life and helping others. It thus appeals to the heightened moral sense of donors but at the same time can be expanded and co-opted for more overtly political purposes (see Copeman 2009b, 2009c).

Donor Stories

Blood donors in Penang came in remarkable variety—men, women, married, unmarried, young or middle-aged, middle-class or working-class, Chinese or Indian Malaysian, Malay, and others. When I asked donors why they had come to donate blood, the replies would often come in the form of the stock phrases employed in public education campaigns and hospital posters, such as "to save a life" or "to help people." Such posters were prominently displayed in blood banks and at other sites of donation, including the mass campaigns that I have described. More persistent questioning could elicit more complex motivations tied to the life stories and kinship relations of donors.

I was interested in how blood donors viewed giving blood and what resonances of kinship or connection one might trace in these acts. One or two donors stood out as being, in the Malaysian context, unusually dislocated from the world of kinship. There was the man described in my opening vignette who enthusiastically recounted his experiences of having donated 104 times in different hospitals in Malaysia but who, when asked about his family, grew quiet and indicated that he was divorced and lived alone. Another, a particularly jovial Buddhist monk in his orange robes, was proud to relate that this was his seventy-sixth donation and that he had already filled up one blood donor's booklet. He told me how "being a monk, saying prayers for people, teaching, and donating blood" were part of what, for him, constituted "a meaningful life." Before becoming a monk, he had worked in a textile factory, but going to work, coming back, and going on holiday had, as he put it, "no meaning." "This is more meaningful," he said, "helping people." When I asked whether he had kept his old blood donation booklet, he chuckled and said, "Yes, it's my passport to heaven—if I have to show it." These—perhaps exceptional—cases indicated how, in a life in which kinship did not fulfill normative social expectations, blood donation might expand to take on a heightened significance.

In a more measured register, other blood donors conveyed how blood donation was entwined with their own kinship stories. One middle-aged donor, whom I met together with her sister at a large blood donation campaign, told me that she had been donating for the previous eight years. When I asked what had first motivated her to donate, she told me that her father had regularly donated blood—he had donated more than one hundred times. When he died, she had decided to begin donating blood herself as a way of honoring his memory. Since then, she had donated twenty-two times. But, she told me, she always donated to the GH (General Hospital) because the other hospitals (meaning the private ones) charged for blood. Other stories revealed further interconnections of kinship and commemoration. Often, donors told me that they had been donating for many years and had first started to donate with members of their family—a father perhaps, or brothers. They had first done this when a family member was ill and needed a blood transfusion but had continued to donate on a regular basis, sometimes with the same companions, sometimes alone. This insertion of blood donation into ties of kinship was visibly demonstrated at many blood donation campaigns I observed, which donors attended accompanied by their spouses and children. Large-scale blood drives were generally held on a Sunday and had the air of a festive day out, with children milling around and the atmosphere enhanced by the food and drink provided for donors and their families.

I was intrigued by the way that the booklet carried by blood donors, which contains a record of the date and location of each donation, could become a material record of the life stories of regular donors. I was shown many such booklets in which a long list of donations meticulously recorded in hospitals and blood donation centers over many years in fact not just traced the events of donation but could be read as the history of a life— where a donor had lived and worked and also the reasons that had dictated donating in a particular hospital, town, or city. Often donors took some time to explain to me the background story of family or employment history to which the list of donations recorded in their donor booklet alluded but left in shadow. Thus, one man in his forties who had come to a hospital blood bank to donate told me that he had donated forty-two times. The first time was in 1985 in Melaka, his hometown. After that, he donated in Ipoh, where

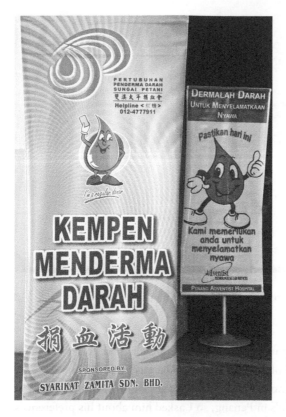

Posters encourage blood donation using "save a life" phrasing.

he had studied engineering, and then in Kulim and Penang, where he subsequently worked. One of the striking things about this donor was that his donor booklet was the original one he had been given in 1985 when he first donated while still in school. The booklet thus constituted a kind of life history of his movements through Malaysia, and his student and working life, with an official verification of each stage provided by the different hospital stamps. He had supplemented this with a checklist of his own at the back of the booklet, giving a tally for each town and hospital and the number of times he had donated there. Different hospitals normally give donors a new donor book, but the medical lab technologist who took his blood told me that some donors prefer to keep just one booklet rather than several. She had some regular donors who had donated more than fifty times. She had

This blood donor booklet records a full history of donation experiences.

taken blood from this donor several times before, she said, and had formed a quite detailed picture of the kind of person he was.

The booklet this donor carried also showed that he had given blood in several different hospitals in Penang, so I asked him about his preferences between these. He told me that he no longer donated at one particular hospital because he had gotten fed up when they rejected him three times in a row because of low hemoglobin levels in his blood. The last time he had told them it was a half-hour journey from his work—and his hemoglobin was only just below the required level. They still didn't take his blood, and so, he said, he had come straight to the blood bank where I met him. Staff there had found his hemoglobin level to be sufficient for donating. "Maybe [they use a] different metrology," he said, suggesting perhaps that efforts to standardize the microprocedures of blood donation are only partially successful. I asked him about how the different hospitals compared. He named another hospital as better "because gives money"—a supermarket voucher for 50 Malaysian ringgit. "So from that point of view, better," he said. "But money doesn't come into my calculation. Do it to help. My contribution.

Also because it's healthy. Feel well afterwards. Get calm, happy feeling. Mentally well."

The same donor mentioned that the General Hospital was less good from another point of view: the procedure of donation was "sometimes painful" there, which he attributed to the staff not using anesthetic. He also told me that he was still scared of the needle, though he had donated so many times. "The technology at GH is less up to date. Hemoglobin check is not the digital one," he said. And he named another hospital where "more people go because of payment. Guess they charge more for blood." He related how he had persuaded two friends from his workplace to donate regularly, telling me that they would send each other emails after they had donated to remind each other to go. These were colleagues, he said; they "used to be my subordinates so I know them quite well." In the past, he had donated once or twice a year, but now he aimed to do so more often and tried to donate in his birthday month. This series of comments from one donor illustrates well how perceptions and judgments of different aspects of donation "bleed" into, and resonate with, each other. This renders the stabilizing project of boundary objects and infrastructures, which I discuss further in the conclusion to this chapter, always contingent.

Several themes emerge from the accounts of the many blood donors I talked to. I have already mentioned the complex interweaving of narratives of blood donation and kinship—and this was highlighted both by the way in which donors attributed their motivation for donating blood to their relations with family members and by practices of donation whereby donors would very often be accompanied by children and other close relatives, some of whom were also donors. The location of large-scale events in a festive and convivial structure heightened the possibilities for resonances of kinship to be enfolded into blood donation. At one mass event organized by a Buddhist association, a hospital blood bank manager described how donors are encouraged to bring their families to "help build family ties" and to "influence family members." Bringing younger members of families and children, he said, "helps to ensure the next generation of blood donors." Another member of staff from a different hospital blood bank added, "Blood is life in Chinese ideas.[2] People who come are working people—that's why they do it on Sundays. Sunday is family day. Seems like a big family." He

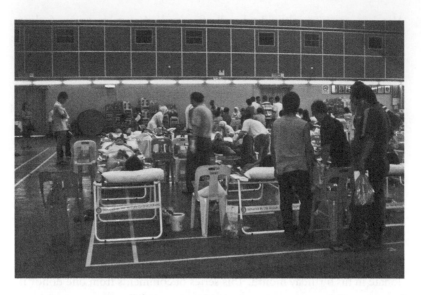

A blood donation drive often brings out repeat donors and their family members.

pointed out how the "aunties are helping. Children can eat too. Meal is not just for donors themselves but also for their families." Emphasizing the fact that the food was vegetarian, he noted how this meant that, "although it's a Buddhist society, Malays and Indians come too. Multiracial society. But all come—no barriers." While donors did not make explicit analogies or metaphorical links between the giving of blood and the importance of blood as a symbolic marker of kinship, it was nevertheless clear that acts of blood donation were already inserted into a nexus of kinship relations or into life stories and narratives of kinship. And the marking of birthdays or the commemoration of particular kin by acts of donation, which were mentioned by some donors, are suggestive of the way such resonances could be amplified in a more personal register.

Donors had preferences and made judgments about different hospitals, mass campaigns, or going to a hospital blood bank on an individual basis. Sometimes this was a matter of convenience, but clearly some donors enjoyed the more sociable aspects of giving at a collective event—the idea that it was "like a party" as one donor expressed it. While almost all talked in terms of "saving a life" or "helping others," and explicitly denied taking

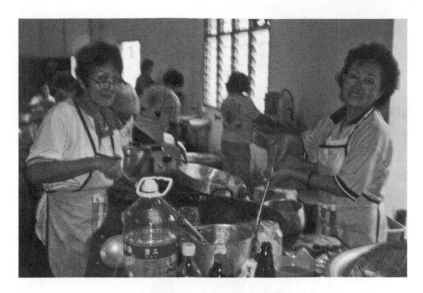

Members of voluntary associations often cook meals for blood donors at large events.

into account the forms of recompense hospitals gave, they often spontaneously spoke about and compared the various gifts or benefits offered by hospitals or mentioned the charges exacted from patients.

Another topic that emerges in some of the narratives I have cited was the belief that blood donation has a beneficial effect on the health of the donor. Many donors told me they liked to donate because it was healthy or mentioned that they felt well after donating. In such views, the regular donation of blood has beneficial effects of cleansing and renewal. These ideas were also articulated in quite similar terms by blood bank staff. One doctor, giving a speech to promote blood donation at a campaign, spoke of various health benefits of giving blood, including that it was "good for the heart. If you give blood three times a year, you have a 50 percent reduced risk of heart attack." Male donors were more common than female donors, and this distinction was often articulated in terms of the idea that, in menstruating, women naturally and regularly shed and replenished their blood, which was believed to be healthy. Male and female donors sometimes spoke about how it was "good for one's health to get rid of old blood and get new," or as one female Malay donor put it, "Good for health to change blood [*ubah darah*]. Good

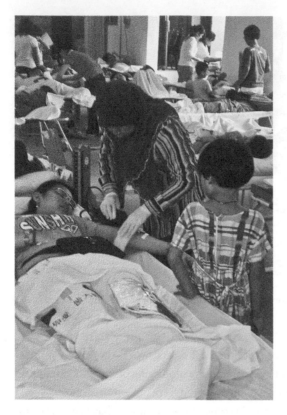

Blood donation and
kinship are often
interrelated.

for health and good for other people." The idea that some of these motivations might merge was made clear by another female donor, a worker
who was donating for the third time at a blood campaign organized at her
factory, who told me she was donating "to help others. Good for system if
you get rid of blood. Will encourage the body to produce more." Although
one might expect discourses about the effects of donating blood on bodily
health to differ for donors of different ethnicities, the Malaysian Chinese,
Malay, and Indian donors I talked to articulated these ideas in markedly
similar terms (see Kuriyama 2002). And this reinforced other statements by
donors, which emphasized their positive valuation of mass blood campaigns
for being multiethnic. Because blood donation encapsulates ideas about
health and illness, commemoration and kinship, personal histories and civic

duty in a particularly dense way, attempts to remove these connotations to produce blood as an objective entity are only partially successful—as I argue in the conclusion to this chapter.

Payments, Charges, and Gifts

One motif that runs through many of the conversations I had with donors is their comparison of different hospitals in terms of the recompense given for blood donation. While most donors said they did not take such matters into account, it is clear from the narratives I have quoted that they were generally aware of the different systems operated by the various local hospitals. Broadly, donors made a distinction between the private hospitals, which gave some kind of gift to donors, and the public General Hospital, where such gifts were not given. Actually, the distinctions between hospitals were more subtle. For example, the blood banks of the private hospitals that I observed had different practices. In one, voluntary blood donors were offered reductions on outpatient charges on a sliding scale depending on how many times they had donated. Thus regular donors were rewarded for their loyalty and commitment in donating blood. Donors were also sent letters of appreciation by the blood bank and, after donating a certain number of times, received a certificate. All donors were given a drink and a sandwich before leaving the blood bank. In another private hospital, voluntary donors received a supermarket voucher for 50 Malaysian ringgit, and replacement donors got a special towel or a polo shirt and a cloth bag. These items were embossed with the name of the hospital and blood bank. Again, all donors were given something to eat and drink before leaving the blood bank.

While I did not observe blood donation at the General Hospital, I was told by blood bank staff from other hospitals that donors there qualified for various benefits, such as being eligible for better wards if they were hospitalized. Although donors never explicitly said they were attending a specific hospital in order to receive a particular reward, it was my impression that, for some donors at least, a supermarket voucher would be a significant addition to their current funds.

At the mass blood campaigns I attended, organized by various voluntary groups, there was an emphasis on nurturing the "helping spirit" of donating,

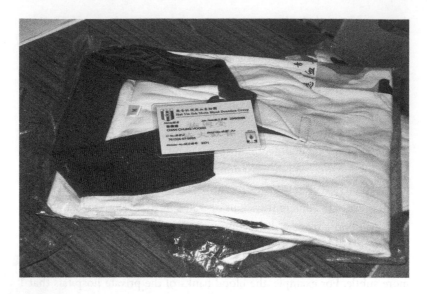

Some events and hospitals offer rewards for donors.

and this was perceived as being embodied in the provision of a communal meal rather than on giving donors any kind of substantial reward. Indeed, I was told on various occasions by the organizers of these events that they did not give gifts to donors. Donors nevertheless received a small bag containing a drink and a sandwich and sometimes small novelties, such as a calendar, a notebook, and mandarin oranges. Regular donors who had given a certain number of times were rewarded by the voluntary organization with certificates, medals (bronze, silver, or gold as appropriate), and sometimes other items, such as a polo shirt, in recognition of the number of times they had donated. It was my impression that donors appreciated these tokens as official recognition for their meritorious acts. One of the largest organizations that I followed held an "Annual Appreciation Day" event for their regular donors, involving a meal and speeches as well as presentations to their outstanding donors. Another held a large-scale charity dinner with entertainment, speeches, and presentations to mark all their fundraising activities. Both of these events included at least one speech made by a local politician, and this underlines the possibilities of such events for political elaboration (see Copeman 2009b, 2009c).

The distinction between the different kinds of rewards offered by hospitals and voluntary organizations is thus less clear-cut than it initially appears, and it touches on other kinds of distinction. I have mentioned that whereas public hospitals in Malaysia took blood only from voluntary donors, following World Health Organization guidelines, private hospitals also operated a replacement system, and they also distinguished replacement donors from voluntary ones in terms of the rewards they gave to donors. Voluntary donors were encouraged not just to donate blood once but to become "regular donors," and as such they might receive various kinds of recognition—from material gifts to certificates and medals, or eligibility for various kinds of health benefits at the hospital where they donated.

Many of the blood donors to whom I spoke voiced a preference for giving blood to the public General Hospital rather than private ones. From the donors' point of view, this preference was articulated in terms of a perception that private hospitals charged patients for blood. Because their blood was freely given, donors often strongly expressed the view that their blood should be given to patients free of charge. However, doctors and blood bank staff at the private hospitals were extremely sensitive to what they clearly saw as a misperception on the part of some donors and the wider public in Malaysia. In their view, this misunderstanding had taken hold because of persistent media misreporting. In fact, blood bank staff explained, the charges to patients for blood transfusions covered the costs of screening, cross-matching, and equipment, all of which were priced. They insisted that these charges did not include any payment for the blood itself.

Perhaps what is significant here is the scope for misunderstanding and the sensitivities aroused. When I gave a talk on my research to doctors at one of the hospitals where I had done research, one of the main points of their questions was how to correct the deleterious public perception that private hospitals charged for blood. Donors, as we have seen, often spoke of their motivations in terms of "helping others," "sharing," "saving a life"— precisely the terms used in publicity to encourage people to donate blood. And similarly, the organizers of the voluntary associations active in recruiting blood donors articulated their ethos as being about "encouraging the spirit of giving," "helping each other," and "helping to build family ties." In their view, the general atmosphere not only encouraged a "family spirit" among donors, nurturing the next generation of donors, but was also intended to strengthen interpersonal ties in society more generally. Some of the donors who came to the blood banks at private hospitals, however, voiced suspicions about such voluntary associations. When I asked whether they ever donated blood at events run by these organizations, some responded that they preferred to give at the hospitals because, when patients needed blood for transfusion, the associations tended to favor their own members. Since blood given for transfusion is under the control of blood banks rather than any voluntary association, this was a misperception. But its resonance is indicative of the tensions between different ideas of what is involved in giving blood and the layers of entanglement of motivations, interpretations, and histories of the institutions involved. That such tensions may be largely hidden was indicated in my opening vignette of two donors, apparently engaged in a similar act but subject to quite different pressures and motivations.

Donors frequently told me that they wanted their blood to go to anyone who needed it. They were particularly against the idea that access to the blood they had freely given might be in some way restricted—either through the levy of charges by hospitals or by the preferential treatment of some special category of patient, such as the members of voluntary associations. Thus the fact that private hospitals charged for the costs associated with transfusion—even though these were carefully calculated to offset the costs of treatment rather than any charge on the blood itself— somehow interfered with perceptions of donated blood as a freely given gift and caused obvious tension. But one might say that such "interference" was already prefigured in the way that blood donation was situated in a complex nexus of expectations surrounding relationships, rewards, costs, and gifts.[3] Donation might strengthen social and civic ties, but it also had the potential to further a mistrust of bureaucratic institutions (see Healy 2006). The various technologies and infrastructures hospitals use to deal with donors and blood that I describe below are thus partly means of holding in check the ever-present possibilities of blood overflowing its boundaries of meaning in ways that might negatively impact on hospital procedures and public perceptions.

Categorizing Donors

During the process of donation, blood comes under the supervision of blood bank staff. In order to initiate this process, a blood donor enrollment form must first be completed and signed by all intending blood donors. This form is a crucial point of mediation between donors, their blood, and its entry into a hospital blood bank through the working practices of blood bank staff. Because different versions of these forms are used by different hospitals, we might consider them an example of what Geoffrey Bowker and Susan Leigh Star call "boundary objects"—"objects that both inhabit several communities of practice and satisfy the informational requirements of each of them" (1999, 16). Such objects, Bowker and Star suggest, have a crucial role in the use of classification and the emergence, maintenance, and control of standards. They "are able both to travel across borders and maintain some sort of constant identity" (16). All of these characteristics are applicable to blood donor enrollment forms, although, as we will see, their efficacy in this respect is at best incomplete. Boundary objects, in the sense deployed by Bowker and Star, work across different communities of practice, and they "have different meanings in different social worlds" (297). Operating across different hospitals and different medical systems (such as the public and the private), blood donor enrollment forms were completed together by donors and blood bank staff. I was interested both in the requirements of the form itself—in other words, the information that donors were required to give—and in the manner in which the forms were completed.

The most obvious difference between these forms was that the public hospital one was monolingual—pointing to the dominance of the Malay language and Malays in multiethnic Malaysia—and required somewhat more detailed responses from both potential donors and blood bank staff. It also included more background information and used tick boxes for negative and positive answers more consistently. The private hospital forms were shorter and were printed in several languages. But apart from these differences, I will highlight some common features of the information they collected and the manner in which these forms were completed.

The blood donor enrollment form enables two important processes to occur. One is the distinction of potential donors from those who are deemed unsuitable or at high risk of passing on infected blood. The other is

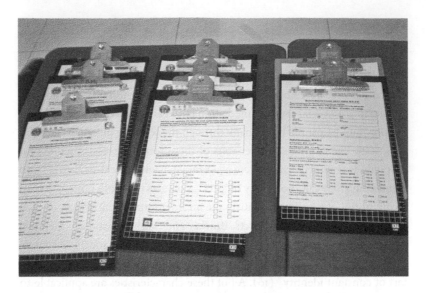

Blood donor forms are printed in different languages.

the provision of information that will enable donors to be traced should the blood bank need to contact them. This might be, for example, because after screening, their blood turns out to be infected, or it might be because it belongs to a rare blood group, which is needed when the supply in the hospital blood bank is inadequate. The forms used by private hospitals distinguished between voluntary and replacement donors. These forms thus provided a link between some hospital patients and some blood donors. The link does not connect the blood of patients and that of specific donors directly because the blood taken from replacement donors was not normally used for the actual patient whose transfusion the donor is replacing, and it may well not be a suitable match for that of the patient. There were, however, some cases in which patients or their family members specified that the blood of family members given as a replacement donation should be used for a transfusion. In almost all cases, however, patients received anonymous blood. But patients in the private hospitals I observed whose family members or associates had "replaced" blood they had used from the hospital blood bank were charged less for their transfusions than those who had not. And blood bank staff members were aware that patients and their families might make a more direct association between blood given to patients in transfusion and replacement blood supplied by family members or others. Thus, in one case I observed in which replacement donors came to the blood bank, they were turned away by blood bank staff, who told me that this was because the patient had a rare blood group, which differed from that of the replacement donors. Because blood is not generally donated directly for the use of particular patients, this was somewhat surprising. The medical lab technologists explained that, because the blood of the donors was not a match for that of the patient, should they subsequently not have a sufficient supply of the rare group to transfuse the patient, they were concerned that the patient's family would be justifiably upset.

Alice Street's (2009) analysis of the intersection of biomedical and kinship (mis)understandings set in place by replacement blood donation in a New Guinea hospital underlines the enhanced potential of replacement donation to feed into local perceptions of relationality and personhood. As she demonstrates, from the standpoint of donors, the hospital itself may then be seen as an "active agent" of extraction and as producing new kinds of relationships from which donors themselves feel excluded—with the negative connotations this implies (Street 2009, 211–12). In the case of Sri Lanka, where the government has attempted to move from replacement/ paid blood donation to voluntary nonremunerated donation, Bob Simpson (2004, 2009) shows how tensions surrounding different kinds of donation and the ambiguities of different meanings and resonances of blood are especially likely to be amplified at times of national crisis. As the Malaysian case underlines, for donors and their families, replacement donation has greater, or more obvious, relational capacities than voluntary blood donation, and this reduces the possibility of it being perceived as an impersonal object. The blood donor enrollment form and other kinds of boundary infrastructure, which aim to objectify blood, constrain but do not eliminate the prospect of such interpersonal and unstable meanings of blood coming to the fore.

I was intrigued by the form questions that had no obvious function in terms of tracing donors or highlighting risk. The first section of the forms, giving personal and contact details, included questions about occupation, marital status, and "race" (*keturunan*). None of these social categories had an obvious connection to the presumed function of the forms. This was supported by the fact that when blood bank staff at one of the private hospital blood banks I observed entered the data on the forms into the blood bank computer system, this information was omitted. The computer data system recorded all the contact details and information about blood grouping, hemoglobin levels, and screening results but did not include details of medical history or other personal information supplied by donors. This could in theory be accessed by going from the blood bank computer back to the donor enrollment form.

When I asked blood bank staff why there was a question about "race" on the forms, they readily admitted that they didn't really know. I sometimes pressed this question since neither the labels on blood bags nor the computerized data in at least one of the blood banks recorded the "race" of donors. It seemed that this was simply a carryover from the public hospital forms. And indeed *all* official forms in Malaysia tend to ask for this information, which is also carried on Malaysian identity cards. The answer is thus prefigured on identity cards and also given by the boxes supplied on the public hospital forms: "Malay, Chinese, Indian, Other (state)." For Malaysian citizens this is a normal part of very many bureaucratic procedures, and the required response is completely familiar.

The Malay term *keturunan*, which is normally rendered as "race" in English, can be more literally translated as "descent," but the English term "race" as well as the Malay *bangsa* are widely used in public discourse in Malaysia in contexts where "ethnicity" might be used in Western English-speaking contexts. Although most local donors thus gave the standard and expected response on their identity cards (i.e., Malay, Chinese, Indian, or a named *orang asli* (aboriginal) group from Sabah, Sarawak, or peninsular Malaysia), when I examined a batch of completed forms for a three-month period at one hospital blood bank, I found a minority had quite surprising answers to this question. Some of these gave a religious affiliation under "race," such as Muslim or Buddhist; others gave a nationality, such as Indonesian or Filipino. The variation was possibly connected to the fact that most private hospitals in Penang have a high proportion of foreign patients (many of whom are from Indonesia). These answers reflect both uncertainty about what was being asked and a conflation of ethnic, "racial," national, and religious categories, which, as noted in the introduction, is a more general feature of public discourses in Malaysia (see also chapters 2 and 4).

Part of my interest in the answers to this question on the blood donor enrollment forms was in case it revealed a link between attitudes toward ethnic origin and ideas about blood. There is a danger of overinterpretation here partly because, as I have emphasized, the answers to this question were largely pre-scripted by what was on donors' identity cards and other widespread bureaucratic norms. More significant perhaps than what was recorded on the forms was the fact that not all hospital blood banks found it necessary to enter this information into their computerized data system.

When I asked blood bank staff about links between these categories and types of blood, they generally said that there was no particular connection, although sometimes a higher frequency of Rhesus-negative blood among Indians was mentioned. Thus, talking to one staff member in a hospital blood bank about why this information was on the form while she was keying information from forms into a computer, I was told that it could perhaps be used to check for a correlation between Rhesus-negative blood and race, "to find higher incidence for Indians" (see also Ong 2016). When I queried whether this would be useful, the conversation turned quickly to more political matters via a discussion of National Blood Centre policies. The issue of educational quotas for Chinese was raised here in negative terms; "We Chinese work very hard," I was told. Talking about the collection of this information thus immediately led to a discussion of stereotyped ethnic categories because, in many contexts in Malaysia, that is what the categories connote. No one working in the blood banks, however, raised with me the possibility of counting donors by ethnic category. But this kind of conversation carried obvious traces of the submerged connections between the donation of blood and ethnic or political categorization.

Some medical lab technologists did tell me anecdotally about particular incidents when they had come across a patient's preferences for blood from donors of a specific origin, making clear at the same time that this was a highly sensitive topic and that it had no bearing on blood bank practices. The idea that Muslims in Malaysia are hesitant to receive blood or organs from non-Muslims has been widely discussed in the Malaysian media and has been combated by the pronouncements of Muslim clerics (see Peletz 2002). Perhaps what is revealed by the collection of this information is mainly the pervasiveness of the categories and the degree to which asking such questions is normalized and unmarked, although, as I have indicated, the issues underlying them are extremely sensitive.

Refusing Donors

Donors would complete their enrollment forms in the reception area of the hospital blood bank in just a few minutes. The medical lab technologist on duty would then go through the answers with the potential donor before taking their blood pressure. Usually, this would be done rather briefly and generally without going through each question separately. The degree of privacy during these conversations varied considerably, but it was often possible for other blood bank staff or donors to overhear such conversations. In one hospital blood bank, a small interview room was used by medical lab technologists for these discussions, and for taking blood pressure and testing hemoglobin level and blood group. Most such conversations were on a one-to-one basis, but sometimes others were present. For example, it was not unusual for several student nurses from the hospital nursing school to come to the blood bank to donate blood together, and they might all crowd into the interview room at once for their tests. In any case, it was my impression that it would be extremely embarrassing for medical lab technologists to ask donors in detail about their sexual behavior or intravenous drug use. And this was confirmed by members of blood bank staff, who said they couldn't really ask male donors if they had ever used prostitutes or about their sexuality, and they just hoped the answers given on the forms were truthful. Thus when I asked one medical lab technologist how she interviewed blood donors and negotiated questions about their sexual behavior, she told me, "Can't ask about sexual behavior—[they] would walk out if [I] asked 'are you gay?' Just assume." She went on to delineate types of donors of whom she wanted to ask such questions, describing with gestures what she saw as a "gay type with earrings. But can't ask." Donors responses to questions were thus supplemented by medical lab technologists' own judgments, assumptions, and experience, as well as by screening procedures.

Staff in the hospital blood banks that I observed took the view that some people came to the blood bank when they already knew they were ill. They did so, I was told, precisely because blood screening procedures for donated blood would reveal certain conditions, such as HIV-positive status, without their having to pay for these tests. A subsequent phone call or letter from the blood bank asking the donor to return to the hospital would confirm to them that something was wrong. Members of staff were united in their condemnation of such behavior, which, in their view, put the health of others (including blood bank staff) at risk. But this of course introduces another hidden aspect of the economies of care enfolded into blood donation procedures, whereby some minimal part of the financial and other costs of positive HIV status that must be borne by patients are mitigated or avoided.

While in most cases turning potential donors away was relatively unproblematic, the care taken by blood bank staff and the reactions of some who had come to donate made clear that this could potentially be a charged process. Often there was some reluctance on the part of donors to accept the verdict of blood bank staff that they were not eligible to donate. One staff member explained to me that "some donors are very stubborn—they want to donate. Have to find a reason to reject them," indicating that this might sometimes be difficult or sensitive. In another case, when a voluntary donor came to donate in the blood bank, the medical lab technologist on duty noticed that he had an eye infection; he was also due for a minor operation. I asked whether she noticed the donor's infection or if he had said something first. She said, "I noticed. When interviewed them, have to look at whole face." Later that morning, this donor was still in the blood donation area with his wife. Colleagues working in the blood bank consulted rather anxiously with each other about him. They explained to me that the donor was upset with the more senior member of staff who had stated that he was not a suitable donor. She said it was "very difficult to reject donors—because of [the] association"—referring to the voluntary association that was active in organizing blood campaigns among regular donors, and which regularly supplied blood to the hospital's blood bank.

These cases illuminate the way that the rejection of donors can be a personal disappointment and is liable to cause offense. Precisely because giving blood is perceived as a moral act, and because the regular donors and voluntary organizations that are vital for ensuring adequate stock at particular hospital blood banks are often embedded in long-term relations, rejection is a fraught issue that may carry pejorative overtones. The boundary work involving forms and judgments about bodily signs, which determine who is eligible to donate, carries moral and political weight. Its exclusionary effects—for example around normative sexuality, HIV status, or racial categories—have been documented in other cultural contexts (Lederer 2008; Seeman 2010; Strong 2009; Weston 2001). Although likely to be handled by blood bank staff with caution, sometimes mitigating these effects, such refusals have repercussions for both staff and donors. And this is heightened when a rejection is enacted in a semipublic context or in front of family members or colleagues. In this way, turning away potential blood donors is a crucial aspect of the social exchanges in which blood donation participates.

Conclusion

I began this chapter with a vignette of two donors lying side by side as they donated blood, whose superficial resemblance was belied by a striking contrast in the motivations that had brought them to the blood bank. In one case, the moral recognition associated with giving blood over several decades seemed to have an expanded significance in relation to a minimal family life; in the other, the obligations of family ties apparently exerted a coercive power. Tracing stories of blood donation has highlighted the complex interweaving of categories, histories, and economies of care that are enfolded into them: judgments about public and private hospitals, and their different—and changing—regimens of practice, made by regular and occasional donors, who may give blood on a voluntary or replacement basis, and who have particular understandings and expectations of the rewards, payments, gifts, and charges in which blood donation is embedded. Even a measurement as apparently neutral as the hemoglobin level can be enfolded by donors into comparative moral judgments about different hospitals and their practices. Further categorizations take place when blood is received in the blood bank: assessments about high-risk donors and about those who are suitable or unsuitable, which are themselves layered into the decisions and attitudes of donors themselves, including their ideas about the effects of donation on their own health. Ethnicity, marital status, family ties, gender, sexuality, and age collide with measures of blood pressure and hemoglobin count, and with screening results for HIV, syphilis, and hepatitis, as well as judgments based on the appearance and behavior of donors made by blood bank staff.

The enrollment forms that donors complete tell their own story of the categories that inform bureaucratic practices, and I suggest that viewing them as "boundary objects" might help to bring their significance into focus. In one sense, we might view blood itself as a kind of boundary object in that, crucially, blood requires standardizing for medical purposes. And this is a consequence and expression of its polyvalent qualities. While Bowker and Star emphasize how boundary objects have a key role in "developing and maintaining coherence across intersecting communities" (1999, 297), we have also seen that categories—such as "race"—on the forms are not necessarily determining or stable and may feed into the relations between blood bank staff and donors in unforeseen ways. As Bowker and Star's work underlines, information systems, or "boundary infrastructures," in institutions such as hospitals bring into communication numerous different social worlds (1999, 313). One might say that the donor enrollment forms are attempts to hold stable the kinds of fluidity of meanings, the "inherent ambiguity" (Bowker and Star 1999, 307), that blood encompasses. In this respect, however, their effects are limited—and these limitations imply that the concept of boundary objects is itself insufficient for the present contexts. Even in the restricted case of the donor enrollment forms, their functioning as boundary objects is highly qualified, and this is because blood itself (as the more plastic object to which the forms refer) condenses too many meanings and resonances to be held stable in the context of donation. Threatening always to overflow its boundaries, blood cannot be contained within the constraints of a boundary object. Conversations with donors revealed the slippages and connections between different aspects and resonances of donation procedures. Decisions to donate are, among other things, also stories of kinship and acts of commemoration, embedded in layers of family relations as well as those between workplace colleagues. We can begin to understand how histories of relatedness and moral, medical, and other categories penetrate each other and are inseparably entangled within acts of blood donation. In the end, as Bowker and Star suggest, classifications that are constructed through boundary infrastructures matter "because they are suffused with ethical and political values" (1999, 321). These intersecting and overlapping meanings also imply that an analysis of technologies can only take us so far in elucidating blood work. The tensions surrounding the refusal of would-be donors—where rejections that may be based on negative judgments by blood bank staff are only reluctantly accepted by those wishing to donate—highlights such limitations.

Veena Das, commenting on the ethnography of "transplant worlds," has noted its "fragmented character" (2000, 284), which she attributes to the different social worlds that technologies of organ transplantation bring together. The observation applies well to the present case where the nature of blood's embeddedness, dispersed as it is across many sites and domains, results in ethnography that is likewise fragmentary. But this dispersal also highlights the polyvalent ethical and moral dimensions of blood donation. Far from being reducible to the morality of a freely given gift, *pace* Titmuss, its polyvalence demands a particularly close attention to the "fine texture of life" (Das 2000, 284) across many different social worlds. This reveals not only that blood donation is entangled with personal biographies, kinship relations, and histories of care—and in this sense is a gift that may also carry Maussian qualities of the person—but also that it has the further capacity to be expanded into political ritual. Alongside the acts of care that blood donation signifies, we have seen more self-interested motivations as well as acts of persuasion—as in my opening vignette. The tensions surrounding the possibility of charges for something freely given, the hidden payments families of patients may make to donors, or the alertness of blood bank staff to the would-be donor who could be seeking confirmation of a suspected illness suggest that economies of care and their objects may be multiple, indirect, and obscured.

The hidden economies of care that blood donation encompasses can also be seen, through another lens, as a hidden politics. Blood donation encompasses the most personal and intimate relations as well as the abstractions of citizenship and nation. It has the capacity to open up issues of trust at familial and institutional and governmental levels. It might then take its place beside more overtly familial practices in anthropological excavations of the paths between politics and kinship. That kinship is understood to be incontrovertibly a repository of moral values (Bloch 1973; Faubion 2001; Fortes 1969; Lambek 2011; McKinley 2001) means that it has a uniquely legitimizing force when it is silently or explicitly evoked in political rhetoric or ritual, and this is intimated too in the comments of participants at larger blood donation events, which I have cited. In this chapter I have paid close attention to the personal motivations of donors and the sense of moral worth they derive from their acts. If we recall that male donors somewhat outnumber female ones, it might be suggested that giving blood endows a sense of self-worth through being a particular kind of virtuous labor that complements both their own paid daily work and women's day-to-day domestic labor.[4]

Donors can equally be construed as citizens of an ethnically plural nation. The act of donation is one possible refraction of civic duty, providing a two-way passage between personal or familial loyalties and national ones. In the contexts I have delineated, blood affords a naturalizing effect whereby the abstractions of nation and citizenship can be understood and made personal. The donor booklet could then be construed as an alternative document of citizenship (the "passport to heaven" of one donor's quip), complementing but also diverging from national passports or identity cards.[5] It records the history of a life in terms of its locations, moral acts, and commemorative practice. As we have seen, donation also asserts differences between citizens and reinforces exclusions within the nation. But the donor booklet as "passport to heaven" also takes us beyond family and discourses of citizenship to an ethical duty redolent of religious ritual, and involving shared substance, that is not anchored in modernity or its institutions—and indeed could be construed as their critique. These kinds of associations do not necessarily need to be articulated; temporally labile, they may be implicitly present in the vial of blood in a lab or in the ideas that bring donors to a blood drive.

At different points in the stories of donation told here, some categories are brought into focus more sharply; others recede. The moral qualities of blood can merge with medical ones or become dissociated from them. Categories and qualities may reinforce each other, or they may screen each other from view. And this raises further questions about the import of such entanglements once blood has entered the blood bank. Following the donation of blood, and its separation into blood products, what shadows are cast by these intense and apparently overdetermined characteristics? To find answers to these questions we need to move further into the world of the blood banks and medical pathology labs and learn about the lives of those who work there.

Before starting work, some of those employed by the clinical pathology labs and blood banks gathered over breakfast. At one hospital, a daily copy of *The Star* would be pored over and passed around; at others, staff members might bring their own newspapers to read during breaks. Items of interest would be commented upon. While, as alluded to in the introduction, political events in Malaysia were unusually exciting in 2008, discussion of politics in the labs was generally muted. Other topics were often more evident in conversations between lab staff. These included the week's supermarket discounts, appliances and electronics on special offer, and advertisements for sales or bargains. They might also be matters about Chinese and other religious festivals, corruption scandals, hospital or medical news, or transportation problems. A few of the medical lab technologists were interested in lottery results. When I asked about this, they showed me where they were printed in the newspapers. From this topic, it seemed obvious to ask how lucky numbers were chosen and about ideas of luck more generally. And following such conversations, I was not surprised to see the headline "Sign Up for 080808 Wedding" in the local section of *The Star*.[1] The article concerned the Penang Chinese Town Hall (PCTH) "targeting 88 couples for its mass wedding on Aug 8." The PCTH secretary was quoted as saying, "080808 is a good date and we hope to attract 88 couples for the ceremony." Such interpolations between items in the newspapers and conversations in the hospitals provided unexpected learning opportunities. As well as conveying the wider Malaysian backdrop against which this ethnography is set, these stories were of the kind that piqued the interest of hospital workers and others whom I encountered.

Fundamentally important for the daily lives of most Malaysians were very large price increases in gasoline, electricity, and gas announced at the beginning of June 2008. As a result of the restructuring of government subsidies, the price of gas for commercial and industrial uses went up by 26 percent and for retailers and small restaurant operators by 18 percent. Gas at the pump went up from RM1.91 to RM2.70 per liter, and diesel from RM1.58 to RM2.58 per liter. The large front-page headline in *The Star* on June 5 read simply, "RM2.70." Other price increases followed swiftly. People everywhere talked about their impact, especially for transportation costs but also for restaurant and hawker stall food charges. The medical lab technologists whose work I was observing worried about using their cars to get to work and began to go out to lunch less frequently. Newspapers in June and July 2008 featured articles on such topics as carpooling by office workers,[2] as well as "Ways to Beat Rising Healthcare Costs."[3] That increasing numbers of patients were turning to public hospitals was also reported. One housewife was quoted as saying, "I may spend more time waiting to see the doctor but I don't mind, especially after the fuel price hike."[4] Those working in the clinical pathology labs of the private hospitals where I was based told me that the numbers of patients had dropped. Newspapers also reported that the government was clamping down on migrant workers from elsewhere in the region and that many would be sent home.

These were serious matters, as were reports about religious topics, which are often politically sensitive in Malaysia. A discussion about whether those who had converted to Islam upon marriage could be allowed to give up Islam following the death of their spouse, if they wished to, was ongoing in connection to one court case. Another widely reported case in the Syariah High Court concerned a former Muslim religious teacher who had become a follower of the Sky Kingdom sect and was convicted in February 2008 of apostasy. A Catholic weekly, *The Herald*, was in dispute with the government over whether the word "Allah" was exclusive to Islam or could be used in non-Muslim publications. Although these cases were of particular concern to academics and human rights activists, I was not aware of them being discussed in the working contexts that I frequented in hospitals or at blood donation campaigns.

Other common news items concerned crime reports—especially robberies and violent crimes both in Malaysia and abroad. Reports about urban gangs and about foreign domestic maids who robbed and attacked their employers were staple fare of local news. Murders, other violent crimes, and serious road accidents were often reported in striking detail, with information about culprits' and victims' personal and family lives. Accompanying photographs would show culprits or victims as well as the scenes of crimes or accidents more graphically than appeared to be the norm in neighboring Singapore's press. Photos of road accident scenes with images of heavy lorries or buses and the concertinaed or compressed cars with which they had collided, debris strewn across the road, and pooled blood visible on the tarmac were not unusual features of such news reports. Here blood would have more violent connotations, and its visual features were graphically displayed to gain the attention of readers. Sometimes reports of road accidents were explicitly connected with donation—as when the organs of a victim of a motorbike accident were used in transplant surgery. Stories intended to have an uplifting message might relate the personal details and circumstances of an accident of the person from whom organs used in transplant surgery had been procured. These details could feature in items about transplant surgery or in those that related the ensuing details of the lives of those who had earlier been the victim of a serious accident. The public life of blood in these stories thus connected violence, both accidental and intended, to personal and family lives, and sometimes transformed its connotations of death, injury, and loss into stories of moral redemption and hope.

There were also many less serious matters—ranging from the humorous to the quirky. There were reports about movie stars, about particular good deeds, about love affairs or family and marital relations. In the state of Terengannu, "a property negotiater" and "father of 25 children" was reported to have "received the blessings of his three wives to wed his newfound sweetheart who is 29 years younger than him." The Syariah High Court approved his application to take a fourth wife under Islamic law.[5] A "25-year-old working girl" wrote to The Star's "Dear Thelma" advice column about problems with her boyfriend. Avowedly content in her work, she described how she had broken off with a previous partner, even though he was close to her family, because of "insecurity in the relationship." She had now found another boyfriend with whom she was happy, but this time there were problems with her family, who, she wrote, "immediately said that he is not the right man for me and I should stay away from him. I couldn't believe this reaction, just because he is of a different race and religion. This has never been a problem for us as we settled the religion issue much earlier." Threatened by her family with disownment, she was searching for a solution, and Thelma responded in forthright terms: "Frankly, if religion and race is the issue with your family, then you should not be held at ransom. We live in a multi-racial, multi-religious country. Mixed marriages have been long accepted. Why would they threaten to disown you on such bigoted terms?"[6] Advising that, "eventually, love crosses the boundaries of colour and religion" and that once the couple were married and had children, her family would accept things, the way forward was made clear. While such accounts do not minimize the power of religion and "race," they also assert in a recognizably Malaysian register that it is possible to transcend the borders these differences apparently create.

Stories like those I have cited about the local economy, discounts or price raises, love matters, accidents, violent crimes, and exotic or unusual events were likely to interest lab staff and be the subject of conversations. They reflect some of the particularity of the Malaysian context at the time of my research. We have seen that this context includes the deep embeddedness of a set of associations encompassing ideas about religion, ethnicity, and what is locally termed "race," and how these may easily become attached to other ideas about appropriate behavior and morality. A certain relish in the details of personal and family matters and in images of violence and blood, which is certainly not restricted to Malaysia, could enhance the interest of readers and give such stories traction. They remind us too that blood can readily be associated with violence and death. Matters such as food, marriage, the family, sexual behavior, and blood and organ donation—or even ideas about vampire spirits, voting preferences, street demonstrations, or luck—may expand the resonance and reach of these associations further. In the following chapters, attending closely to the details of "blood work," the people who perform it, and the sites where it occurs enable us to understand better the myriad ways in which such matters seep into lab processes—as well as the "boundary work" that attempts to ensure the separations between the labs and the world outside.

TWO

Lab Spaces and People

Categories and Distinctions at Work

Give me a laboratory, and I will raise the world.
—BRUNO LATOUR, "Give Me a Laboratory and I Will Raise the World"

Decorative fish tanks were not high on the list of what I expected to find when I embarked on fieldwork in the clinical pathology labs and blood banks in Penang's hospitals. But they were present in several of the sites I observed. Some were professionally made displays of tropical fish for the benefit of patients. Others were more obviously homemade ponds, seemed to be a hobby for staff, and were fashioned from disused containers. These ponds and plants had a distinctly homely air and might be located at the back of a set of clinical pathology labs between various backrooms. They made a radical contrast with the bright, air-conditioned labs with their up-to-date artifacts of modern medical technology. These ponds, as I learned, had been constructed and were maintained by some of the lab staff in their spare time.

In the summer of 2012, while revisiting one of the labs where I had worked previously, I was intrigued to find that staff had rather mixed feelings about their sparkling new premises, with its closed-off work areas, its glossy, manufactured aquarium with fish, and its clearly marked boundaries regulating public access. Several complained that they no longer had a view of the outside world from the lab windows, or that they couldn't see their colleagues while working as easily as they had done in the old place. One medical lab technologist said that the previous premises had been "more like a house, more friendly." The new lab was bigger, which necessitated more walking; things were "very separate," and doing on-call duties at night was now more frightening: "Can't hear if someone comes, like in the old place—could hear everything." Another told me, "The new lab is a *real* lab," and I thought he was about to expand on its advantages in positive terms. But instead, he referred to the fact that it felt more like a workspace and that blood donors liked it less because of the "hospital atmosphere."

●　●　●

There are different ways of entering the blood banks and clinical pathology labs. Like many houses, they have more than one point of access—front doors and back doors as it were. And like houses, which door one uses signifies (Carsten 1997). This is partly a matter of familiarity. One entrance was generally reserved for patients, another might be for blood donors. A different door (perhaps to the rear of the others) was only for staff. Visitors who belonged to none of these categories seemed to know which entrance was appropriate for their use. The fishponds described above were part of the "backstage" of one set of clinical pathology labs. They were not visible to patients or other outside visitors, just as the labor that went into maintaining them—that of male members of staff on weekends and in their free time—was also "invisible" lab work. The area where they were located could be accessed directly by staff; from here, one could go into the labs through the back door.

　　The connections between people, the spaces they inhabit, and the processes in which they engage are crucial to many ethnographic studies. In this chapter, I introduce the staff of the clinical pathology labs and blood banks, and I describe the spaces in which they work. We begin to discern how boundaries operate in the labs—the ambiguous manner in which these spaces constitute a world apart and yet also replicate life outside the labs. Paying attention to social categories in the labs, we see how gender, kinship, and ethnicity permeate these spaces. In this sense, the sociality that is enacted here takes recognizably Malaysian forms and emerges from familial and personal histories, "histories in person" (Holland and Lave 2001), that have been shaped by the wider political and social history of Malaysia, particularly in the latter part of the twentieth century. Part of what is distinctive about the labs and blood banks occurs through the intertwining of ethnic diversity and gender in ways that are molded too by the specificity of

Penang within the cultural geography of Malaysia. As I intimated in the introduction, the work that goes on in the labs also requires a separation from the outside world, a process of purification in the Latourian sense (Latour 1993). Here fishponds, at least those of the professionally manufactured kind, might speak to images of containment and the sealed-off nature of these labs. But the more homemade variety with which I began this chapter suggests a more compromised laboratory space where processes of domestication can also be detected. The maintenance of boundaries is a necessary aspect of the spatiality of the labs and has material expressions (Bowker and Star 1999). This might be true of any laboratory space. What difference does it make that these are labs that are centrally concerned with blood and other bodily samples? As we saw in the previous chapter, the many meanings of blood evident in donation stories make it particularly resistant to becoming a stable "purified" object. I suggest that the marking of boundaries and their simultaneous permeability in these spaces is especially problematic because of the blood and other bodily materials derived from donors and patients that are the focus of lab work.

We have already encountered the pervasiveness of ethnic categories and stereotypes in Malaysia. This pervasiveness also extends to the labs. Here ethnicity may have negative connotations; but diversity is also actively welcomed—and we might see this too as a recognizably Malaysian phenomenon associated with contemporary urban life. Enfolded within ethnic, gender, and kinship typologies are more specific personality types that could be seen as particularly suited to the requirements of laboratory life. The work of the labs seems to thrive on a synergy between a stance of engaged sociability and one of quiet, serious reserve. While the latter might be more readily associated with laboratory diligence, I show how both types together (as well as their intermediaries) contribute to successful outcomes in these hybrid laboratory/clinical sites.

Just as there are many ways to approach the blood banks and clinical pathology labs, there are different categories of people who do so. Patients and blood donors may have reasons to visit these sites, but their access is restricted to specific areas, and they are not permitted to wander freely in the labs. Then there are the occasional visitors: nurses from other parts of the hospital collecting bags of blood for transfusion; engineers from medical technology firms engaged in maintenance or repair of the sophisticated diagnostic machinery; sales reps from such firms; computer support staff from inside the hospital, or from outside, who maintain the complex data information systems of the labs; dispatch staff taking or delivering samples between different labs or between departments of the hospital; staff from the hospital stores delivering supplies; and hospital maintenance workers fixing problems with the air-conditioning or performing other routine repairs. These are just some of the people who might have reasons to pass through the labs and blood banks. Some might pay more "social" calls or combine a working reason with a more sociable visit. Former colleagues as well as staff from elsewhere in the hospital might also drop by just on a friendly basis.

But the main inhabitants of the blood banks and clinical pathology labs were not the occasional visitors but those who actually worked there. They included the receptionists and clerical staff, cleaners, dispatch staff, the lab manager, and, most important of all, those responsible for running the many diagnostic tests in the labs as well as the day-to-day work of the blood banks—the medical lab technologists and lab technicians. Numerically and structurally, the medical lab technologists were at the center of what went on in these spaces. Much of what I describe in this chapter and those that follow focuses on these social actors and the work with which they engaged.

Before introducing the main protagonists, I begin with a description of the spaces they inhabit. Just as the house space defines and is also shaped by the interactions between its inhabitants and that of visitors (Allerton 2013; Carsten and Hugh-Jones 1995), so too the working spaces of the labs and blood banks both circumscribe the activities of their occupants and can be subject to creative adaptations—the fishponds being a striking example. The labs and blood banks of different hospitals varied in size and in the number of staff they employed, and this affected their spatial layout, the work they were equipped to do, and the organization of tasks between staff. Here I amalgamate some of their features to highlight their most salient social characteristics.

Spaces and Boundaries

Clinical pathology labs and blood banks were clearly bounded spaces with controlled access points. Doors were marked "No Entry," and one could not mistake the fact that these were not public spaces. They were separated from blood donation areas or areas where hospital outpatients had blood or other samples taken. The labs were divided into departments for different kinds of tests: biochemistry, immunology, hematology, serology, urinalysis, bacteriology (or microbiology). Bigger sets of labs had more departments, including, for example, cytopathology and histopathology. In most cases, these departments had two or perhaps three people working together in them. Although different departments occupied particular areas and had equipment (including some large pieces of diagnostic machinery) associated with their tests, the most striking feature of the spatial layout of these labs was that, internally, most departments were easily accessible to each other. With a few exceptions, described below, the departments were not closed off from each other by walls and doors. The spaces were free-flowing, so that one could easily walk between them and see what was going on in different part of the labs. Since the same samples or equipment might be used for different tests, and colleagues might need to consult each other over specific results, accessibility was a necessary feature of the different departments. Of course, it also had social correlates. Colleagues could easily walk over to a different part of the lab for a quick chat when there was a lull in the work. They could also help each other out at times of high pressure. Work patterns were highly visible to colleagues and to the lab manager or others passing through. From an ethnographer's point of view, the spatial layout of these labs was advantageous because, from most departments of the lab, I could easily see what was happening in other areas and move between them without formality when something interesting appeared to be happening elsewhere. On the whole, these were spaces of quiet sociability, and both the nature of the work and the layout encouraged easy social interaction between colleagues working in the same or nearby departments.

While the main departments of the lab flowed into each other, and people worked at their benches, sinks, centrifuges, diagnostic machinery, microscopes, and computers for data entry in quite close proximity, some areas were more self-contained than others. The microbiology (or bacteriology) departments were in separate rooms with their own fume cupboards, sinks, and refrigerators for storing petri dishes, in which bacteriological samples were being grown on agar jelly. The doors to these departments were, for health and safety reasons, supposed to be kept shut, but those who were working inside were visible from other areas of the lab through

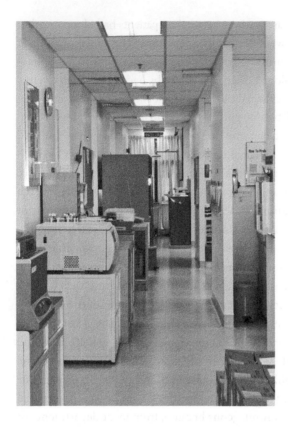

The spaces of the lab with their equipment are orderly and high-tech.

windows or glass doors. The lab managers had their own offices that opened onto the main areas of the labs, but the doors to these were normally open and often the lab manager would be elsewhere—taking blood from outpatients, working in one of the other departments of the lab, or sometimes at a management meeting in the hospital. If the lab hierarchy included a consultant pathologist, she too would have a separate office—the door in this case generally shut—and a secretary located outside. The histopathology and cytopathology labs associated with the consultant were also quite self-contained departments that operated behind closed doors but were nevertheless accessible to staff in the rest of the lab and visible through windows and glass doors.

The blood banks came under the same management as the labs and formed part of the same spatial units. They were partially self-contained

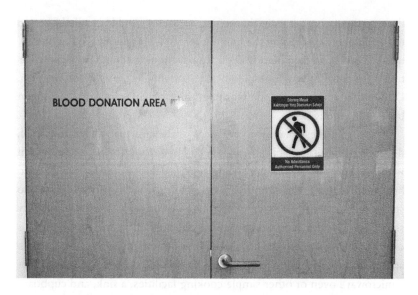

Blood donation areas are one of many lab spaces where access is restricted.

spaces within the larger clinical pathology departments. The blood banks consisted of interconnecting areas—one with seats for the reception of donors, a space for the screening of donors, and an area with several beds for donors who were giving blood. They had their own centrifuges, refrigerators and freezers for storing blood products, other equipment, and a computer for recording data on donors. Usually, two or three of the lab staff were assigned to work in the blood bank. The blood banks had their own entrances for donors and other visitors leading to a reception area, but on smaller premises this might also be the main access for visitors to the labs. Doorways for staff, but not for donors or patients, led between the blood bank and the main departments of the lab.

The other large working area of the clinical pathology departments was an outpatients' section where patients referred by doctors from the hospital outpatient clinics for blood tests came to have their blood taken. Like the blood banks, these were to some degree self-contained sections that communicated with the other parts of the labs. Staff could come and go easily between these areas, but patients did not enter the main working areas of the lab. They reported to a reception desk where a receptionist would direct them to the rows of seats in the waiting area, and would be called forward to the phlebotomy area by the member of staff who had picked up the request form to take their blood. Medical lab technologists and lab technicians trained in phlebotomy took blood from patients in the phlebotomy area. During the busy hours of the morning, the lab managers could also often be found working here.

Apart from these main working areas of the labs that I have described, depending on the available space, there might be a dedicated meeting room with a center table and chairs. In addition, "backroom" areas were used to house storerooms, cleaning rooms or areas, and toilets. There were also spaces for the use of staff when they were not on duty. These were clearly separated from the main working areas, screened off at one end of the labs or in a space adjacent to the main labs. They housed tables and chairs where staff could eat and drink, a fridge for food, a kettle for making drinks, perhaps a microwave oven or other simple cooking facilities, a sink, and cupboard space or shelves where staff could keep their own mugs and plates. I have already mentioned how the staff of one set of labs had made their external off-duty area pleasant with plants and fishponds. The facilities for staff might also include an on-call room with a bed and a small shower room so that staff could stay overnight or rest during a lunch hour.

The most prominent sign of differentiation in these spaces was the clearly marked boundary between the labs and the rest of the hospitals of which they were part. Lab staff and patients used different entrances to the labs and blood banks. The entrances used by staff were clearly marked "Staff only" or "No entrance, authorised personnel only." Other working visitors might choose between these, but nurses and other familiar visitors to the lab would usually use the same entrance as the lab staff. On occasions when the CEO of the hospital was showing important visitors around the lab facilities, he would bring them through the "front door"—the same one that patients and blood donors used. The second important point is the relative permeability of space within the lab. Lab staff would move between the different departments (which were not necessarily very clearly demarcated) quite freely, and doing so was encouraged by the lack of physical barriers. The firmly shut door of the consultant pathologist created one reserved zone, but by contrast, the door to the office of the lab manager tended to

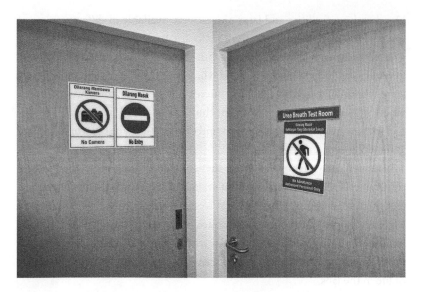

Restricted access contributes to the boundaries of the lab.

remain open, and people would go in and out of it with minimal ceremony. In this way, the labs formed interlocking areas of hierarchy and familiarity.

Another clear principle by which space was divided was according to whether it was a working area of the lab or an area used by staff when they were off-duty. Work and leisure were for the most part spatially separated from each other. But this distinction operated in conjunction with another important marker of spatial zones—hygiene. When food was eaten together at work, it was either in the area with tables and chairs or, if this was too small, in a meeting room that was a designated "clean" zone—where no diagnostic testing took place and where no blood or other patient samples were present. Hygiene was a fundamental concern for staff who worked in the labs and blood banks, and food was not allowed in the main working areas. As I describe in chapter 4, this did not, however, mean that it was not an important part of social relations between colleagues.

As might be expected in working spaces that routinely involved dealing with blood, sputum, stool, and urine samples, concerns about hygiene were visibly manifested—and are discussed further in the chapters that follow.

Handwashing facilities and latex gloves were available in different areas of the labs and blood banks, as were sinks for handwashing in the off-duty spaces. These were extensively used, but there was also quite a lot of variation between individuals in how and when they used latex gloves while they were working (see chapter 3). The microbiology department was one area where particular caution was taken; this was reflected in the way this department was separated from others and the fact that lab staff working there generally wore face masks.

Many of the variations between the labs that I observed seemed to be a result of differences in management style and structure. These affected not just the spatial layout of the labs and working practices but also qualitative aspects of social relations between colleagues. Thus quite small distinctions in how labs were run, or the particular working style of a lab manager or another key figure, could make a significant impact on many different aspects of life in the labs.

The use of space in the labs was not fixed and unchangeable. On the contrary, whenever I left the labs for a few weeks or months—or sometimes even days—I was struck by some change that had appeared in the meantime. These were often small adjustments in the layout of equipment or how particular areas or benches were arranged. When I revisited one set of labs after an absence of about eight months, staff pointed out major acquisitions in diagnostic machinery, which had necessitated rearrangements in spatial layout. So the increasing importance of biomedical technology in this line of work affected how space was used, and often a new piece of biomedical machinery meant the introduction of a more mechanized, or more up-to-date, procedure. Observing a series of reconfigurations of layout in different labs, I perceived an evolution of spatial forms such that the boundaries of the lab and their division of internal space became more marked as technological sophistication increased. As can be deduced from my introductory vignettes, for those who work in these spaces, technological innovations may be ambivalently received.

Changes in personnel, by contrast, could generally be accommodated within existing arrangements of space. In one set of labs, there was a member of staff who took particular care organizing how the equipment in the labs was arranged and initiated frequent small changes in the layout of apparatus or minor improvements to furnishings that were intended to make the work go more smoothly or to improve safety, hygiene, or convenience. Colleagues generally accepted these with good humor, and sometimes joked about the parallels between this person's fastidiousness at work in the lab and his own home, where, according to his wife, it was equally hard to keep track of the constant rearrangements of furnishings.

As I have noted, the seniority of people who worked in the lab was less obviously reflected in strict demarcations of space than might be the case in many other working environments. Medical lab technologists would use the tables and chairs for eating together with clerical and secretarial staff, and these spaces might also at the same time be used by some cleaning staff and by the lab managers—although there were differences between sets of labs in practices of conviviality. Gender was even less prominent than seniority as a spatial organizing principle. Staff of both sexes seemed to work easily alongside each other and also used the same off-duty facilities, including lavatories. But as I elaborate below, gender was a noticeable principle in the employment hierarchy of the lab.

Along with the work inquiries, test tubes with blood or urine samples, paperwork, and items of lab equipment, other kinds of knowledge and information moved easily between work benches and sections. During busy times, especially in the mornings, these might be restricted to quite brief questions about home life, family members, or social events. Prospective outings or meals involving lab staff were always a favorite topic for conversation. Planning that day's lunch or inquiring where a colleague was going for lunch were likewise matters of interest. If work pressures were less intense, then longer conversations might be possible—about films, outings, children, staff in other departments of the hospital, or recent social activities. Since many of the staff were women with young children, they often swapped information about children's illnesses, vaccinations, and treatments for minor ailments, or discussed sleeping patterns, schools, clothing, and other matters of concern surrounding their children or other family members. Newspaper and other media stories were also likely to feature in conversations between lab staff. The first months of 2008 were a period of quite intense political upheaval in Malaysia. Newspapers were sometimes present in the lab, and they generated a steady but generally fairly understated commentary about the election campaign and results of the general elections held in March 2008 and other major news stories. Prominent as topics for discussion were media reports of sudden price hikes following the withdrawal of government subsidies on gasoline, local political scandals, reports on criminal activity, discount sales, lottery results, and the like.

Many of the visitors to the labs were familiar figures—and some, like the engineers who came to fix occasional problems with biotech machinery, were not only regulars but also a channel of communication between lab staff working in different hospitals on the island. They often did a little double-take on seeing me one day in one hospital and then on a different day in another. These visitors would swap news and jokes with regular staff, sometimes showing pictures on their cell phones, exchanging gossip, or participating in a meal. Other, more occasional visitors were former members of staff who came to visit their colleagues and spouses or parents of staff who had come to the hospital to see a doctor or for a diagnostic test. In the following chapter I pursue some of the ways in which the world outside the lab penetrates the working environment of the lab, but here I focus on the characteristics and attributes of those who work in the clinical pathology labs and blood banks.

Whether they were housed in separate buildings or located in the main buildings of a hospital, the clinical pathology labs and blood banks formed distinct departments with their own management structure. Partly because of the nature of the work of medical lab technologists and their specific training, partly because the labs were spatially set off from other areas of the hospital, and partly because they had their own managers (who were in turn responsible to someone else in the hospital hierarchy), the labs had a strong ethos of their own. The medical lab technologists took pride in doing their work well, which they articulated in terms of the speed and accuracy of their results, and had a strong sense of loyalty to their colleagues. They often spoke of the hospital management in wry or somewhat cynical terms and were particularly suspicious of attempts to increase their workloads or change their shift arrangements. The job of the lab managers could involve quite delicate balancing between the demands made by the hospital management and the needs and preferences of lab staff. A preferred lab manager from the lab staff's point of view was one who was seen as capable of standing up for their interests in the face of increasing workload demands from the hospital management. To the extent that the labs were at least partially separate zones, with their own habits of sociality, this fostered a sense of corporate solidarity within the labs. Such a feeling was articulated in the comments about lab premises in my opening vignette, which record a sense of nostalgia for old labs that were "more like a house, more friendly."

Introducing the Lab Staff

The main work in the different departments—carrying out diagnostic tests on samples, taking blood from patients and from blood donors, separating donated blood into blood products, cross-matching blood for transfusion— was carried out by medical lab technologists and (to a lesser extent) by lab technicians. Whereas the medical lab technologists had a degree in a science subject (such as biology, chemistry, biochemistry, genetics) or a degree or diploma in medical lab technology, followed by practical training in the labs, the lab technicians had no university education and had been trained on the job in the labs. Depending on how long they had worked in the labs and their level of training, the lab technicians were restricted to a narrower range of tasks than the medical lab technologists. This usually included phlebotomy and might extend to some of the diagnostic tests. Some of the lab technicians I encountered had only recently left school, while others had been working for several decades in the labs and had been promoted to senior lab technician. In the labs that I observed, there were just two or three lab technicians, and about ten to twenty medical lab technologists. The latter were by far the most numerous category of staff in the labs.

The lab managers that I encountered were in their fifties. They had worked in the labs for many years, sometimes having begun their careers in a different hospital. After leaving school, and perhaps after holding one or two other jobs for a few months, they had found work in a hospital, for example in a clerical capacity or as a lab technician. Following training in medical lab technology and working as a medical lab technologist for a number of years, they had been promoted to lab manager. Some had had periods working as a medical lab technologist or lab manager at another hospital. While they might be older and more experienced than some of the medical lab technologists, their training and career backgrounds were essentially similar. And some of the medical lab technologists and lab managers had been colleagues for several decades.

The other personnel working in the labs were support staff—including clerical workers, receptionists, secretaries, cashiers, dispatch officers, and cleaners. The number of people employed in these capacities varied depending on the size of the lab. A smallish lab might have just one or two receptionists, a dispatch officer with no other clerical workers, and no cashier. Payments would be handled by the hospital cashier's department, and cleaning would be part of the hospital housekeeping department. A larger lab would need more support staff and have its own cashier and its own cleaning staff.

The medical lab technologists were both the most numerous category of personnel and, in terms of the work carried out in these spaces, the core staff. Most of my time in the labs was spent tracking the medical lab technologists, observing them and talking to them about their work and their lives more generally. By extension, I was also interested in the lab managers who supervised this work and were responsible for the day-to-day running of the labs and blood banks, and in the lab technicians who performed some of the same tasks alongside the medical lab technologists. These three categories could be seen as stages along one career path. Lab managers could start out as lab technicians and become medical lab technologists before being promoted to managers. But of course not all medical lab technologists expected or wanted to become lab managers. And not all had started as lab technicians. Equally, some lab technicians never became medical lab technologists—although if they stayed in their jobs for many years, they might expect to become senior lab technicians.

These observations give rise to some questions: How does one enter this career path? What kinds of people, from what kinds of backgrounds, take up this career? What kinds of education and aspirations do they have? Perhaps most importantly, what do these stories have to tell us sociologically about contemporary Malaysia? This last question may be answered in many different ways, and I return to it at different points in the following chapters and in the conclusion. The more time I spent in the labs and blood banks, the more it seemed to me that the spaces and the trajectories of staff encapsulated many of the social processes that have marked Malaysia over the last several decades. The spaces were quintessentially modern and "high-tech"; the profiles of staff in terms of age, gender, and ethnicity were obviously varied; some but not all of the staff held university degrees in science subjects. And yet, one could not say that the "modernity" in evidence here had been eviscerated of recognizably Malaysian forms of sociality encompassing kinship, gender, care, and domestication. And so, both from the point of view of the work that went on in the labs and blood banks and from a wider perspective of the sociology of Malaysia, the stories of the lab personnel were of interest.

Age, Gender, and Education

What broad social categories can we discern among lab personnel, and how do they connect to wider patterns of gender, class, ethnicity, education, and social mobility in Malaysia? Staff in the labs were varied in terms of age—for some this was a first job after leaving school; others were in their fifties and nearing the standard age of retirement in Malaysia of fifty-five. The youngest of the medical lab technologists were in their twenties—having completed a degree course—but most were in their thirties or older. The majority of staff in the labs were women—and this was true of both the medical lab technologists and the support staff. Among the medical lab technologists, although the proportions differed between labs, women heavily outnumbered men. The lab technicians (who were far fewer in number than the medical lab technologists) were more evenly balanced between men and women. But all the receptionists, secretaries, and cashiers and almost all the cleaning staff were women of varied ages. The dispatch officers were young men.

Very few of the lab staff were unmarried, and most of those who were married had children. With just a few exceptions, most of the unmarried staff were still young, and some had fiancé(e)s and were intending to marry in the not too distant future. Among the medical lab technologists, as among the other staff, the norm was to be married with children. The largest group of medical lab technologists were in fact married women in their thirties with young children. Born in the 1970s, they would have finished their schooling in the early to mid-1990s.

The overwhelming majority of the lab staff were originally from Penang, and many had elderly parents and other relatives, apart from their conjugal families, still living there. Just a few had been brought up in one of the towns in the nearby northern states of the peninsula. In all of these respects, the profiles of lab staff could be said to be broadly homogeneous, but in other respects their stories were more mixed. I was especially interested in how education and class background played into the career trajectories of lab staff. From the discussion in previous chapters, we could expect ethnicity to be important too. I probed these matters through a set of interviews with members of lab staff (concentrating mostly on the medical lab technologists, lab technicians, and lab managers) in which I asked about their education and training, their career paths, and their family backgrounds.

The most obvious difference between categories of staff was in their levels of education. The majority of medical lab technologists and lab managers held a university degree in a science subject or in medical lab technology or had a three-year diploma in medical laboratory technology from a local institution. Support staff, including lab technicians, did not have degrees. However, a few of the lab technicians and secretaries came to the lab with a two-year diploma from a local private college. A substantial number of the medical lab technologists and lab managers had begun their careers in the hospital as lab technicians, or had at some earlier stage been a lab technician, and had then taken the opportunity to be supported by the hospital to take a three- or four-year training in medical lab technology. This required a period of several years' bonded labor at the hospital on their return. In one hospital, more than half the medical lab technologists that I interviewed had been financed during their training in this way; in another the proportion was much smaller. It was clear that, for those who could not afford to study or who were worried about getting a stable job, this had been an opportunity to acquire qualifications that would lead to secure employment. In this way, the training and career opportunities offered were comparable to nursing.

The importance to career paths of acquiring degree-level qualifications, and the different ways this could be achieved, led me to ask about the parental backgrounds of lab staff. Here the most stark finding was that very few of the lab staff I interviewed had a parent who had been to university. In the great majority of cases, the parents of the lab staff had not been educated beyond secondary school. A number of those I interviewed told me that either one or both parents had only received primary school education. A few said their parents had not been to school at all because schooling was disrupted during the wartime Japanese occupation of Malaya or because their parents had come as immigrants from China.

The occupations of parents (many of whom were retired) were quite varied, but in general they were working-class or white-collar workers. Some had worked in factories or as food hawkers, market sellers, or middlemen; others were clerical or sales staff. A smaller minority had been teachers, accountants, or nurses, and a few had their own businesses. In the majority of cases it seemed that the acquisition by their offspring of degree-level training in a science subject and a secure job in the hospital was a substantial step up in class and employment terms.

Another clear shift from one generation to the next was in the employment of married women. Only a small minority of lab staff told me that their mothers had worked after marriage. In one or two cases a father had died or was absent, and it had been financially necessary for a mother to work in a factory or as a food hawker. In a few other cases a mother had worked as a teacher or nurse. As the majority of staff in the lab were married women with children, this represented quite a big social change from their own mothers' experiences. This accords with national trends that show an increase in women's participation in the labor force from 37.2 percent in 1970 to 47.9 percent in 2011 (tan and Ng 2014, 350).[1]

Some of those I interviewed spontaneously commented on how the era in which their parents had grown up had affected the latter's educational and employment opportunities. Some of the parents' schooling had been disrupted by wartime or curtailed by poverty. When I asked one medical lab technologist whose own training had been funded by his hospital if his parents had had education beyond secondary school, he responded that his father had finished secondary school, but this was in the 1950s and not many people at that time went to university. The profiles of family background and educational histories that I collected very clearly indicated a widening of opportunity and access to education for the current working generation compared to that of their parents. And one could see how this transition was inscribed on the histories of families in the course of the 1950s to the 1990s. Almost all of the more senior medical lab technologists whom I interviewed, born between the late 1950s and early 1960s, stood out as being the only members of their sibling groups who went to university. But for many of those who were born in the 1970s, the situation was more mixed, and even if their parents had had no tertiary education, several of their siblings had been to college or university.

That this was not necessarily a smooth story of upward mobility was underlined for me by one lab technician. Born in the late 1970s, he was the son of retired teachers, and his father was one of the few parents of his cohort who had attended university. On finishing school, the lab technician had gone to a private college to study. But, as he related to me, this was the period of the Asian economic crisis, and when he left college in 1998 with a diploma in engineering, he couldn't find a job. After a short period working in a factory, he had found employment at the hospital as a lab technician. And while working, he had continued on a degree course as a part-time student for a further period.

Mahathir's Children

I have suggested that the backgrounds of lab staff could be taken as reflecting the post-independence, twentieth-century history of Malaysia, with a notable widening of educational and employment opportunities for the local population in the latter part of the twentieth century. But the era in which the majority of the lab staff grew up had another important defining feature. Many who were born in the 1970s finished their schooling in the late 1980s or during the 1990s. Their education thus coincided with the government of Malaysia's longest-reigning Prime Minister, Dr. Mahathir bin Mohamad, from 1981 to 2003. This was mainly a period of political stability and, for many, of increasing economic prosperity.

Prime Minister Mahathir strongly promoted the idea of Malaysia as a modern, technocratic nation, in which the latest technological and scientific advances would be a path to economic growth through development and prosperity. The country's economic objectives were set out in a series of four-year "Malaysia Plans."[2] The expansion of tertiary education and a widening of educational opportunities, particularly for Malays, was an essential part of these processes. In 1991, Mahathir set out his "Vision 2020" (Wawasan 2020) for Malaysia, which avowedly sought to transcend ethnic divisions through the promotion of one "Bangsa Malaysia" (Malaysian race or nationality). Under the plans implemented as part of Vision 2020, Malaysia would take its place among the "fully developed" nations by 2020 on the basis of a combination of hypermodern technology, infrastructural projects, its vibrant economy, social mobility, and its adherence to what Mahathir saw as the fundamental bedrock of "Asian values." A commitment to religion and family life that was explicitly in stark contrast to what he perceived as the decadence of Western societies was central to Mahathir's vision.[3]

Coming from the early post-independence generations of Malaysians who, without being from elite backgrounds, gained access to university education (particularly in science subjects), the lab staff who held degrees or diplomas could be seen as representative of the expansion of educational opportunity and the spirit of development that Mahathir promoted. In this respect, the fact that very few of their parents had been to university and that many were from working-class backgrounds is telling. In other ways, however, government policies might also have significantly constrained their chances, and here ethnicity enters the picture.

The majority of the staff in the labs was ethnic Chinese with a minority of Indian Malaysians and Malays. As Megha Amrith (2013, 236) reports for hospitals in Singapore, both staff and patients came from diverse ethnic backgrounds, and conversations in the labs were multilingual. In the hospitals, the official lingua franca was English, but conversations among staff, or between staff and patients, might be in Mandarin, Hokkien, Cantonese, Bahasa (Malay), English, Tamil, or a mixture of several of these. Other languages also sometimes cropped up, and it was not at all unusual for conversations to take place in two or more languages. Across the labs that I observed, ethnic Chinese outnumbered staff of all other ethnicities by about four to one among the medical lab technologists and lab managers. In Malaysia, as elsewhere, ethnicity also carries connotations of religion (see introduction to this volume). Malays, the majority population in the country as a whole, are Muslim. Most ethnic Chinese are Buddhist or Christian. The majority of ethnic Indians are Hindu and a minority are Muslim or Christian. The preponderance of Chinese Malaysians in the labs (of whom some were Buddhist and some were Christian) can partly be taken as a reflection of the demographic profile of Penang, where, unlike in other Malaysian states, ethnic Chinese are in the majority, followed by Malays and Indians (see introduction).[4]

In order to advance the interests of the Malay population and, in particular, the rural peasant sector, and to further economic development, Mahathir's government introduced policies to promote Malays in the establishment of businesses and in education. The adoption of ethnic quotas for university entrance from 1979 to 2002, and subsequently a "merit" system based on different examination results, made it significantly easier for Malays to enter public universities. University entrance for non-Malays in general required better results than for Malays.[5] When I questioned lab staff about the choices that had led them to their particular careers, several indicated that, had they been less constrained, they might have studied a different subject at university. Some said that they had originally wanted to study medicine; others mentioned that, had it been possible, they would have liked to pursue research in a science subject after their first degree. While some of those I talked to articulated the constraints that had shaped their trajectories quite clearly, these issues touched on sensitive topics about which non-Malays in Malaysia are often hesitant to speak openly. One residue of these policies was the generally high caliber of staff in the labs, their liveliness and talents, and the sense that many who worked there had the potential for more creative or intellectually demanding work if the opportunities had been available.

As I describe in the following chapter, much of the work that is carried out in the clinical pathology labs and blood banks, while highly skilled, is also very routinized. Although some short courses to learn about new technologies were offered to staff, their work was quite repetitive and usually did not require much creative or innovative input. Career development opportunities for medical lab technologists were also limited. In one set of labs the grade of senior medical lab technologist had recently been introduced. But opportunities for promotion or for transfer to other labs were limited. Not everyone could become a lab manager—and it was far from clear that many would want to. Many of the responsibilities of the lab manager's role were perceived as irksome by more junior staff. One or two medical lab technologists who seemed rather dissatisfied with their positions explained that applying to different labs elsewhere in Penang was problematic because of connections between the human resource managers and between the lab managers of different hospitals. Managers might talk to each other and would soon discover if their staff were trying to change jobs. Poaching other managers' staff was frowned upon in a context in which the different labs relied on each other's services or resources, and it was seen as important to maintain friendly relations between them. So some staff members felt stuck where they were and seemed to have few options for career advancement.

Probing Gender and Ethnicity

The features of staff that I have described raise further questions in terms of gaining a deeper understanding of the world of the labs. What lies behind the broad features of age, gender, ethnicity, and educational attainment? Going beyond demographic categories, what *kinds* of people work in these labs? And what implications might this have for the work processes that go on there? How do seemingly pervasive features of the Malaysian social landscape, such as gender and ethnicity, play out in these spaces?

One morning in the lab, I asked Shanthi, one of the medical lab technologists, busy at the time carrying out blood chemistry tests, whether she thought lab work was more suited to men or women. "Women more than men," was her immediate response. When I asked why, she said, "Because more passive." She paused. "But need men too." "In the world, or in the lab?" I asked. She laughed and said, "Both. Actually, lab is our world. Lab is a small world." Later that morning, I asked a colleague of Shanthi's, who was working nearby, the same question. Again I was told, "Women. Men need more challenging jobs. Guys shouldn't stick here. No chance for promotion." She named one of her colleagues who, she said, had been working in the same lab for thirty years. "That's why majority of lab staff is female. In education too—teaching. We're more patient. . . . Construction field mainly male—under hot sun." Then, referring to these attitudes, she said, "Just typical ones. . . . Hospitals—usually caring side is female—nurses. Doctors—male. Now getting more male nurses."

Some of the lab workers I asked agreed with Shanthi and her colleague that women were better suited to the kind of work that went on in the lab— which was detailed and repetitive but at the same time demanded a high level of patience, skill, and accuracy. The topic was brought up spontaneously one day by Kay Jin, a married man in his thirties who had been working as a medical lab technologist for about ten years. Doing a lunchtime stint in the blood bank to relieve another colleague, Kay Jin told me that work in the lab was "ladies' work." When I asked what he meant, he said it was being "an operator on machines." In the past, he said, the tests used to be more manual. He also worked part-time selling insurance, he told me, and wanted to get out of lab work; he was worried about his health. At first I thought his worries were about the possibility of contracting infectious diseases in the lab. But it turned out that he was more concerned about the chemical reagents routinely in use. Kay Jin told me about two friends of his working in the labs of another hospital in Penang, one of whom, he said, had gotten cancer from the chemicals. Maybe the Chinese were more susceptible, he speculated. He said that previously he hadn't been worried, but now that he was a married man he felt he had more responsibilities.

Opinions about the gendering of lab work were not, however, necessarily so predictable or so stereotyped. When I asked another of the medical lab technologists whether she thought lab work was better suited to men or women, she told me quite brusquely that it was not particularly suited to either men or women. "Depends. Some men don't like it because it's not challenging enough. Too routine. Some like it." A more senior medical lab technologist in a different lab said it depended on the person. He went on to describe how early every morning he would check around the whole lab, "To see who's leaving the place properly. We had one guy, Indian, always disappeared. He was a smoker, would go off for a smoke. Could never find him when people phoned. Very irritating." He also told me about another colleague who had now moved to a different hospital where the staff in the lab were mainly men. "But she doesn't like it—most of tests are done manually. She went there because the salary was higher." He had told her before she left, he said, that salary was not the most important thing.

Others agreed that there were more important matters than gender in what made someone suitable for lab work. When I asked another medical lab technologist, Eng Swee, about this, she said, "We need both. But can't have big-headed, choleric types because nowhere to go. We have MLTs [medical lab technologists], senior MLTs, lab manager, scientific officers."

She emphasized that the career development possibilities in the lab were extremely limited, so there was not much to offer those who were highly ambitious. Another of the medical lab technologists whom I asked paused before saying, "More suitable for women maybe? Because more patient. Men more rough, more careless. Maybe gender stereotypes? But manager can be a man." Or a woman? I asked. "Yes, or woman." "But," she pointed out, "mechanical staff—all engineers who do servicing—all men." In some of the other hospitals, she said, there were more men working. "Like postmen— over here [in Malaysia] no women."

So, along with gender stereotyping, these answers refer to various different kinds of attributes that are seen as qualifications for work in the lab. Patience, accuracy, and a lack of overreaching ambition were seen as appropriate characteristics for medical lab technology work, and some staff readily associated these qualities with women rather than men. But many were also quick to question a hasty association between gender and particular attributes, saying that above all it "depends on the person" and their attitudes toward work. And this too was in keeping with their own experience, backgrounds, and career trajectories. Many staff members had themselves surmounted aspects of their own class background and wider expectations about gender in achieving tertiary education in science and making their careers. Both by training and through experience, they had reasons to adopt an open-minded attitude to expectations about gendered behavior.

When I asked a lab manager what he looked for when choosing new staff, he said, "Number one, qualifications. Two, personality—whether helpful enough." The ability to work as part of a team was often emphasized as essential to making the labs run smoothly. The nature of the work tasks and timings—with frequent points of high pressure in some sections—meant it was highly advantageous to have colleagues who were willing to help each other before being asked to do so. Lab staff frequently told me that one of the things they most disliked about their work was receiving calls from doctors or nurses to ask for results that were not yet ready. Where they got on less well with each other or were reluctant to help out, work proceeded less smoothly and delays in getting test results were more likely, which resulted in more phone calls and complaints from doctors.

The almost imperceptible elision from gender to a casual remark about being Indian or Chinese—"one guy, Indian," who "always disappeared"— or a progression from the discussion of gendered skills to the idea that the Chinese might be more susceptible to the carcinogenic risks of chemical reagents, such as those I have quoted here, is an everyday occurrence in Malaysia, where ethnic categories are a pervasive feature of the social landscape. The labs and blood banks, like the wider hospital settings of which they are part, are multiethnic working environments. As in many modern urban contexts in Malaysia, ethnicity (often referred to as "race" in English or "bangsa" in Malay) was part of the background to work and social life in the labs, but one couldn't necessarily predict whether or how it would matter to what went on there. We have seen from newspaper accounts how public discourses about blood and organ donation make reference to ethnicity—if only to vociferously deny its importance or to suggest that ethnic barriers may be surmounted. And in chapter 1 I described how blood donors are routinely categorized by ethnic background, although it is not clear why this occurs. These two features of blood donation are indicative of the way ethnic categories are deployed in Malaysia. That is, they reflect both their apparent inescapability and the heightened sensitivities that surround them. Ethnicity may be a proxy for race, nationality, religion, dialect, or communal group, and all of these may be essentialized and naturalized.

As A. B. Shamsul (1996) and Shamsul and S. M. Athi (2014) have argued, there are not just many levels of ethnic categories in Malaysia, which have a deep historical embeddedness dating back to colonial times, but it is also possible to distinguish an "authority-defined" from an "everyday-defined" reality of ethnic ascription. The former, they suggest, is reproduced textually, for example, through bureaucratic procedures, census categories, reports, books, and academic media; the latter is more personal and is replicated orally in patterns of everyday conversation and practices of sociability. Shamsul and Athi rightly emphasize, however, that these two forms are strongly connected (2014, 268–69). In the labs and blood banks one could "do ethnicity" in a seemingly conscious and/or "authority-defined" way (for example, by filling in forms or generating statistics or reports on lab or blood bank activities) but also "undo" it just as visibly by stating categorically that when it comes to donating blood or organs, ethnicity is irrelevant. The effects of either move are not obvious—though might in fact be similar. I was intrigued by how ethnicity might play out among the staff in the labs and blood banks who were working in areas apparently close to these concerns. Was it, for example, possible simply to ignore ethnicity altogether? Or were there ways in which these social categories reappeared or penetrated laboratory practices?

There are no simple answers to these questions—partly because this is a subject of some delicacy. As already noted, in Malaysia, as elsewhere, ethnicity often codes for language and also for religion. Religious connotations are thus implicitly part of conversations about ethnicity. Working relations between colleagues were on the whole amiable, or where they were not, this was not obviously expressed in a register of ethnic difference. As is common in Malaysia, different cultural practices, cuisines, weddings, funerary rites, and other such matters came up in conversation and were discussed with animation and interest. Relations between colleagues often involved teasing; joking was a ubiquitous feature of working life. When a senior member of staff found fault with someone's work, this was often expressed in a joking manner—especially if it was a relatively minor matter—with a kind of exaggerated scolding. Quite often this made reference to supposed ethnic differences over matters of hygiene or work. Joking allowed room for saying the unsayable and also gave space for a comeback—which was almost always forthcoming. Such banter was particularly prevalent in one of the labs I studied. Sometimes one sensed that an unspoken line had been crossed and perhaps offense had been taken. But impressions could be somewhat misleading unless one knew something about the backgrounds of staff or the history of their relations. There was a complex layering and double-edged quality to this kind of repartee—perhaps the person doing the scolding was himself married to someone from a different ethnic group or had reversed some conventional stereotype about gender; perhaps the spouse of one person was close friends with the other, and so they were on more friendly terms than one might assume.

Apart from a recognizably Malaysian joking register, direct references to qualities or attributes in association with ethnic categories did not occur frequently. Sometimes one of the medical lab technologists commented on the hardworking character of Chinese Malaysians in comparison to other groups; almost always they explicitly or implicitly excluded their Malay or Indian colleagues from such generalizations (see also M. Amrith [2013] on similar processes of stereotyping among nurses in Singapore). I wondered whether ethnicity might make a difference in preferences when selecting new colleagues. It did, but not in the way I might have expected. When new colleagues were being appointed, their ethnicity was always a matter of overt interest among the staff, but the explicit preference—about which there was broad agreement—was to *increase* ethnic diversity. This was because the preponderance of Chinese Malaysians in the labs led to problems over shifts and holidays, especially during the period of Chinese New Year, when too many people wanted to take the same holidays and some were obliged to be available for work. Here a pragmatic valuation of ethnic difference was of greater significance than any predictable preference for ethnic similarity. We might see this as part of a contemporary Malaysian sensibility in which pluralism is an inherent part of the urban social landscape that tends to be underplayed in both popular and academic renditions (see Baxstrom 2008, 2014; Yeoh 2014c).

So far, I have discussed a kind of conscious categorizing or association of qualities and characteristics with ethnic markers that went on in the lab as it does more generally in everyday life in Malaysia. As I have intimated, some of these processes are fairly obvious, while others appear only in subtle or submerged ways. But how might blood enter this picture? What difference, if any, does it make that the specific focus of lab work was on bodily materials, and particularly blood? At various points it was possible to observe the samples that circulated in the lab participating in the connections that might be made between ethnicity, nationality, contagion, and risk. As I was tracking their work, medical lab technologists or lab technicians would sometimes explain something to me in ethnic or national terms: there were higher rates of Rhesus-negative blood among Indians than among other groups, I was told, or most of the positive HIV tests were from Indonesian patients.[6] And of course categorization could occur through an absence, rather than overtly through obvious association. On one occasion, one of the lab trainees, Newton, appeared in the blood bank wearing safety goggles. This was unusual enough for a more senior medical lab technologist working in the blood bank to remark on it. Newton explained that on the previous day he'd had an accident in another part of the lab and gotten blood in his eye. Had he checked the status of the patient, he was asked. Newton said he thought it was a diabetic man aged eighty-two—implying there was no risk involved. Had the blood been screened? No. At this point the medical lab technologist jokingly suggested praying. My impression was that while these kinds of connections might not be overtly made, they were nevertheless present below the surface and could readily be drawn.

One morning, I asked one of the more senior lab staff about a new group of trainees who had just arrived in the lab. He explained the system by which the lab takes on trainees in batches at different times of the year. "At the moment," he said, "we have seven—four Chinese, two Malay, one Indian." Thinking about this exchange later, I was struck by the way ethnic categories here were deployed as a way of counting, as one might say, "five women and two men." But at the same time, this points to how marking ethnic identity is so pervasive that, paradoxically, it comes to have an unmarked quality. Attributing ethnicity is in this way part of the background noise of the working environment. And it is difficult to say whether this is a conscious or unconscious activity or what its implications might be. Returning to the questions with which I began, one could not say that ethnic categories were ignored or irrelevant in the labs. Rather, such categories, and the essentializations on which they rest, seemed almost imperceptibly to permeate most corners of life there. But ethnic differences were also an accepted and in some respects positively received feature of this social world.

Laboratory Types?

As I got to know the staff in the labs, I thought perhaps I could detect some broad personality types that seemed to recur in different sites and different hospitals. Struck as I was by the quiet, cool, and calm atmosphere in the labs (especially when compared to urban street life in the public spaces of Penang), my attention was first drawn to some of the steady, serious, and more reserved members of staff in the labs, who, it seemed, embodied the skills and attributes of medical lab technologists.

Wai Khay was a married woman in her mid-thirties, soft-spoken, very intelligent, and extremely hardworking. When I asked her about the main responsibilities of her job, she listed them: "Making sure sample is taken from correct patient. Running tests, getting accurate results; knowing how to compare results. Having the knowledge background to read results."

In response to my question of what she liked most about her work, she said simply, "The lab environment." I asked her how she had originally gotten into this kind of work, and she told me, "When I was a child I liked the hospital environment. When doing training, thought of working in hospital. Don't know why. Would like to do medical research—maybe academic. Medical interests. Prefer lab work—don't have to deal with people."

In fact Wai Khay often emphasized that what she liked about the lab was the possibility of just getting on with the work, and that she didn't particularly enjoy the "people parts" of her job—dealing with patients or doctors. Nevertheless, when she was going around the wards collecting blood samples from patients, I sometimes observed how they appreciated her quiet efficiency, and in one or two cases, where patients had been in the hospital for a while or had been readmitted, she had obviously gotten to know them and would ask after their families or their health problems. Over time, we developed a kind of teasing relationship over the fact that she strongly maintained that the work of the lab and life outside the lab were quite separate. Wai Khay enjoyed the separation between work and family life: "Some people are more sociable," she told me, "others of us just do our work." When something came up that seemed to call into question this conceptual separation between the world of the lab and the world outside, we would sometimes catch each other's eye and smile. And she did tell me that her closest friends were among her colleagues in the lab, and it was not unusual for her to go out with them after work for a meal or some entertainment.

Emily was another quiet and efficient worker. Also in her thirties, and married with children, she had first come to work in the hospital straight from school about fifteen years before I encountered her. She had then been financed by the hospital to get a three-year diploma in medical lab technology before returning to the hospital to work out her five-year bond. When I asked her to describe her working day, she said, "Start work already. Make sure some reagents working properly; previous day's work is cleared—our turnaround—no dilly dallying. Serology is like that. Work, work. Some departments not." And it was true that Emily was generally to be found hard at work at her lab bench or taking blood from outpatients in the phlebotomy section. When I asked her how she had first gotten into lab work, she told me, "Even in my schooldays I *loved* lab work. Dad is a science teacher. I'm an introvert type. Like to be in the background, not extrovert. Like to be behind the scenes. Some of my colleagues are more extrovert. Don't know why they decide to stay." I asked whether her choice of career had to do with her father's influence. She replied, "He let me decide. Just wished I can find a stable job and a good future."

Like Wai Khay, Emily was absolutely clear about what she liked most in her job: "Most enjoy—keep myself occupied, busy. I love my work. Just not dealing with patients, doctors—very stressful. . . . Very stressful. Would have left earlier otherwise—if I didn't love it." And again, when I asked Emily about how she saw the relation between her home and her working life, she was adamant about their separation: "Always classify them separately—otherwise stressful. At work I'm fully committed to work, don't think about family. At home, switch off work."

Nevertheless, when she spoke about her family, it seemed that perhaps there were some connections between her home and working life. She had mentioned her father's work as a science teacher when talking about her choice of career; her brother, it turned out, worked in a nonmedical capacity at the same hospital as she did. She had another relative interested in studying science who had asked about working in the lab, and Emily had told her she could come to have a look around the lab if she was interested; and a further one was intending to go into nursing and had inquired about the hospital. There is perhaps nothing specific to Malaysia in the way these familial and work connections played out. But highly competent, thoughtful, and quiet as Emily was, I was intrigued rather than immediately convinced by her emphatic assertion of boundaries between work and family life.

We might think of Emily or Wai Khay as "typical" lab workers—somewhat reserved, quiet people who tended to concentrate hard on their work tasks, and who said that they didn't particularly enjoy dealing with patients or the hospital doctors. As I spent more time in the labs, however, I perceived another type among the medical lab technologists who, it seemed to me, had almost the opposite qualities. These were more obviously sociable people who had been attracted to their field of work by precisely those things that others found problematic and who particularly liked working in a hospital setting.

Cheng Suat was about thirty when I met her. Brought up in George Town, Penang, she lived with her natal family and was engaged to be married. She was fluent in several Chinese languages and English and had a three-year degree in science from a university in Kuala Lumpur. Cheng Suat had been working as a medical lab technologist for several years. When I asked what had first drawn her to her field of work, she told me how, after her degree, she had gone for a period of practical training at another hospital. "Was comfortable during training. . . . Went for an interview in a factory, not comfortable." She also said that she had a cousin working in the hospital administration who "called me and asked whether wanted job. Said they need people immediately. Straight away asked me to come. . . . Had already met [the lab manager] during training." Cheng Suat explained that she was already familiar with the hospital. She herself, as well as her grandmother and great-grandmother, had been patients there in the past. "So, quite familiar with hospital. During training, felt not really frightened of blood. Some people get frightened, but to me, feels normal."

When I asked her about the responsibilities of her work, Cheng Suat said, "Have to be very concentrated. Very careful. Double-check. Try to help colleagues in other departments. Most interrelated. Do a bit more, makes rest of work go smoothly." But what she most enjoyed about her work, she said, was "when I see very sick patient, I draw blood, they say, 'Oh not painful at all. Thank you.' And whatever I can help with patients—keeps me in hospital." Cheng Suat emphasized that she liked to help patients who are sick and that she had wanted to work in a hospital. At school she had wanted to do nursing, she said, but her father had discouraged her. "If [I] can help people, very happy."

Others too had a similarly "sociable" orientation in their working lives and found working in a hospital integral to their job satisfaction. Miss Tan (an older and more senior member of lab staff who was usually referred to with a title) was a married woman in her forties with children. She herself was the youngest of a large sibling group. She told me that most of her brothers had gone into business, most of her sisters were housewives, and only one brother had gone to university. She herself had taken a four-year degree in sciences and had been working at the hospital for many years. When I asked her how she had gotten into her present line of work, Miss Tan said, "My course is relevant to medical line. People. Hospital is something like service to community." Talking about what she enjoyed in her work, she said, "I've found it's not boring compared to office work. Can communicate with patients on ward."

Like almost all her colleagues, Miss Tan told me that members of her family tended to ask her about medical matters. And when I asked her whether she saw her home life as being connected to her working life, she responded, "A bit connected. Daughter is in science stream." She paused, and then, suddenly animated, she said,

Each person has a field they go [into]; some more successful, others work very hard, not successful. Same work—why? Born with that type of area to go to. Chinese people believe date and time born—astrology—determines. When small I went to see a man [a Chinese fortune teller], he told me to go into hospital line. He was right.

I was struck by how Miss Tan posed this as a question to me—how could one account for such differences in outcomes between people? And did I believe some people's field was predetermined at birth? I asked whether she thought this kind of aptitude was inherited from parents; she said she didn't and that also it was not acquired through learning. This was a matter of fate.

Miss Tan was by no means the only medical lab technologist to bring up ideas about fate, astrology, or luck when discussing her working life (see also M. Amrith 2013). As we will see in chapters 3 and 4, these matters cropped up unexpectedly in different contexts. But I was somewhat surprised, given her background and training, at her ready attribution of success in her work to astrological causes rather than diligence, learned skills, or even inherited characteristics.

Mr. Yeoh was another senior figure in the lab who mentioned luck in reference to his career choice and his personal relations. In his mid-forties and engaged to be married, he had also been born and brought up in George Town, Penang. After leaving school, he had held a variety of short-term jobs. When I asked Mr. Yeoh how he had decided to go into his current job, he gave an expansive answer:

First thing, by luck. Quit from college. [I became a] lab technician—not bad. . . . They sent me for training—five years right time to decide. Compared with government job, here keep in touch with patients; know if better now. . . . Advise staff to treat patients like family members—take responsibility. Treat every sample as [from] your family when doing blood tests. This is most enjoyable. Not because of salary—can get higher pay in other jobs. Work load not [good]; get tired, but don't feel bored. Not just a job.

Although Mr. Yeoh apparently felt that he had come to be where he was more or less by luck, what also stands out here is a commitment to patients at the center of his attitude to his work—which, notably, he phrased in the language of kinship. This commitment encompasses both the highs and lows of patient care and dealing with difficult results or bad prognoses. In chapter 3 we will see how other medical lab technologists mentioned that dealing with particularly difficult diagnostic puzzles until eventually they reached a definitive diagnosis had given them special satisfaction.

Like quite a number of other lab staff, Mr. Yeoh had medical connections inside and outside the hospital. His niece was a nurse and, partly because he had been working at the hospital for a long time, she had met most of his colleagues in the lab. Mr. Yeoh's fiancée was also a nurse and worked in the hospital. When I asked how they had met, he told me how colleagues in the hospital had tried to find him a suitable partner. This had worked "like magic"—"a matter of timing," he said, and "fate also." Others in the lab told me that there had been several attempts to find a match for Mr. Yeoh, but it had taken some time to find the right person. I think most would have concurred with him that "fate" or even "magic" had a role to play in such matters. Mr. Yeoh was by no means exceptional in having connections of various kinds within and beyond the lab, or in seeing the patients as central to his motivation to do his job well and in imagining connections to patients in terms of kinship.

I have suggested that we can delineate two broad types of "typical" lab staff: the more introverted, "techie" ones who particularly enjoy working in a lab, and those who are more gregarious and socially expansive, and also more obviously committed to working in a hospital environment. Rather than one or other, a mixture of *both* these types together, with their contrastive characteristics, is well-suited to the world of the lab. The complementarities between them ensure the smooth functioning of the labs and the quality of their work.

Although the dichotomy I have sketched is appealing, there are some lab staff who fall less easily into either category. On the whole, these could be described as more detached from the work of the labs. Thus one staff member described how she had gotten bored after being there for some time, and how "guys don't like to stay because they don't have prospects." Another, when asked about her working day, told me, "I'm working. No surprises. Every day, same old thing. Very routine. Sometimes get peculiar bacteria. Quite boring but it suits me. I'm not a very adventurous person." Then, changing her tone abruptly, she began to tell me that she felt that her whole life was based around work. She worked a six-and-a-half-day week: "Work occupies a lot of my life. I used to have a boyfriend." For this medical lab technologist, an expanded work life filled long hours, and her social existence revolved around work too. She was at the center of a network of friendships among the unmarried lab staff or those living separately from their spouses. And she was one of several medical lab technologists who told me of the obstacles to changing jobs to another hospital in Penang because the interconnections between the staff at different hospitals meant that it was impossible to keep knowledge about employment changes secret.

When I asked another staff member whether her parents had concerns about her working in the lab—over safety or worries about contagion—she told me, "Not so much. They're quite happy I'm working here. They will tell people I'm working here in hospital [i.e., with pride]. Tell people I'm a doctor; ask me to advise people."

This kind of pride or satisfaction on the part of parents was mentioned by a number of others when I asked whether their parents worried about them working in the lab, and was also connected to the fact that relatives of hospital workers were eligible for medical treatment at discounted rates. Many of those I talked to explained that their parents didn't really understand all that much about the work of the lab. But unease about lab work as "dirty" was revealed in the ambivalence of some relatives' attitudes toward lab work, as well as concerns of staff about safety in their workplace. These attitudes, which are explored further in chapter 4, indicate how the nature of the diagnostic work carried out in these labs, and the blood and other bodily materials that circulate there, make it particularly difficult to secure the sealed boundaries of the lab space.

Conclusion

I began this chapter by focusing on the marked boundaries of the labs and some seemingly odd juxtapositions in spatial arrangements—between the rather clinical and technologically advanced equipment in the labs and some carefully laid-out decorative fishponds just outside them, bordered by abundant plants. The fishponds alerted me to the fact that the spaces of the lab were not just working areas but also social spaces. Redolent of containment but also of movement and flow, the fishponds visually articulate the ambiguity of the spaces of the labs, which we have seen are both strongly bounded and yet also internally permeable and at least partially porous to the outside.[7] The fishponds also speak of the cooperative effort that is required to maintain them and of the sociable spirit of the lab work I observed—and that is characteristic of Malaysian sociality more generally. Like the blood donor booklets introduced in the previous chapter, the ponds both express and occlude hidden histories of care and of labor, of containment and flow. Redolent of work and leisure, neither wild nor tame, they suggest control of a provisional kind and a domestication that does not rest on a strict separation between home and work. In many respects separated from the hospitals of which they are part, and inaccessible to members of the public, the labs hold a strong sense of corporateness. We have seen how the paradoxically bounded and yet simultaneously freeflowing and permeable spaces within the working areas of the labs are an expression both of the routines of work and of a sense of homogeneity among staff, where differences of seniority (or age, gender, or ethnicity) tend to be overridden by a spirit of cooperation. "House-like" yet also unfamiliar, technologized and risky, the connotations of the lab spaces, which are simultaneously alien and domesticized, are pursued further in chapter 4.

Considering the spaces and people of the labs has apparently inexorably drawn us away from the central topic of this book—blood. I have suggested, however, that the fact that work in these labs focuses on blood and other bodily samples affects the nature of the boundaries of the labs and blood banks and the difficulties of maintaining these. The boundary work that goes on here and the efforts to seal off these lab spaces from the world outside are made particularly difficult by the fact that the work is not, for example, a matter of inorganic chemistry or other nonhuman materials. While there is a strong sense that these working spaces should be sealed off from other areas of the hospital and are not open to the public, the blood and other bodily materials on which lab work concentrates derive from patients or donors, some of whom are known to staff. The many meanings of blood, which are evident in donation, and the social relationships of donors and patients cannot simply be expunged from these spaces—a story that will be continued in the chapters that follow.

We have also seen how the social and educational backgrounds of lab staff and their career trajectories reflect twentieth-century Malaysian history and the policies of successive governments. The rapid modernization projects promoted by Prime Minister Mahathir, the widening of educational opportunities for working-class and middle-class Malaysians, social mobility, relative economic prosperity, and the expansion of full-time work for married women are part of the story behind this particular laboratory life. One important aspect of this distinctive Malaysian quality involves a historically situated entanglement of ideas about ethnicity with the practicalities of educational achievement and employment opportunities.

In describing their education and career trajectories to me, some lab staff conveyed a sense of having been limited or constrained in their choices in the past or of being somewhat bored or dissatisfied in the present. One of the most striking features of life in the labs and blood banks was the obvious talent and intelligence of the people who worked there. Had the opportunities been available, many might have made successful careers in research or medicine. And I suggested that this lack of opportunities might be connected both to government education policies favoring Malays and to the class and economic backgrounds of lab staff. The superabundance of talent—perhaps also referenced by nonwork activities in the labs or the decorative embellishments to those spaces (such as the fishponds)—left a sense that much of the creative and innovative resources of the staff was left untapped by their work.

I have delineated, too, certain types of people who are drawn to medical lab technology: those who are good at science, who like the lab as a working environment; those who prefer to have "not many people to face" in their working life; and those who, by contrast, find something positive in their sociable interactions with colleagues and patients and derive their satisfaction from helping with medical treatment. The complementarity between these types produces a distinctive working environment and enhances the quality of work in the labs. As with any typology, there are those who seem to fit uneasily into these categories and in whom we can discern a mixture of all sets of characteristics. Certain qualities—such as patience, accuracy, a lack of ambition—are regarded as appropriate for the work of medical lab technology. But we have also seen, perhaps less predictably, that fate and luck, as well as pollution and danger, have a role to play in the course that working lives take. And kinship has appeared as a significant trope through which patients and their tests are apprehended—as well as being more literally present in the form of the relatives of staff who come to the hospital for treatment or who are colleagues employed elsewhere in the hospital.

The categories that are most pervasive in the Malaysian social landscape make their presence felt in the lab—and indeed cannot be evaded. Kinship, gender, and ethnicity are lenses through which lab staff perceive themselves and each other. This does not mean, however, that any one of these—or all of them together—would be sufficient to explain the workings of the lab. These are mostly matters that are kept in the background. Ethnicity has a paradoxical essentiality in that it is both asserted and negated; it may be referred to through jokes or negative stereotyping but also, as articulated in newspaper accounts and other public discourse, played down. Partly for pragmatic reasons, but perhaps also for the variety and interest it lends to work routines, diversity in the labs is on the whole welcomed by immediate colleagues. I have endeavored to capture here the quiet, fragmented, everyday sort of knowledge about colleagues, their backgrounds, and their families and the taken-for-granted ways in which it permeates the life and work of the lab. Thus, when Shanthi told me that lab work was more suited to women than men, and added hastily "but we need men too," she revealed the significance of gender to the work processes of the lab but also pointed to the subtleties of the social processes that go on there.

Latour has argued that "the distinction between the inside and the outside of the laboratory is . . . misleading" (1983, 151). What goes on inside, he suggests, is in fact a "displacement" of the outside (154). When I repeated Shanthi's statement, "the lab is our world," to a medical lab technologist in a different hospital, he immediately acknowledged its aptness and also at once made his own amendment: "Yes. A world of our own." The phrase "the lab is our world" is ambiguous. It conjures up an image of a laboratory world that *replicates* the processes of the world outside and also one that is *separate* from what goes on there. Here the sense conveyed in my opening vignette that these lab spaces carry protective and sociable qualities that make them house-like, which are particularly valued by the inhabitants of the labs, is important. Houses of course can be experienced both as sheltering havens and as reproducing the hierarchies, distinctions, and dangers of the world outside. In the chapters that follow we will see that both these aspects of the labs are pertinent. To understand how each matters, and the tensions between them, following Latour's suggestion, we need "to study *the very content* of what is being done inside the laboratories" (1983, 159, emphasis in original). There are of course different ways of following his prescription. We have begun to see how domestication, kinship, gender, feminization, and care (themes that are not prominent in Latour's work) imprint themselves on the labs in particularly Malaysian ways. In the following chapter, I focus on the work processes of the labs and the bodily samples that circulate there in order to grasp more clearly the significance of the boundaries between the lab and the external world and of the obstacles that surround containment.

On Friday, July 18, 2008, the front-page headline of the *New Straits Times* (Malaysia's foremost pro-government English-language newspaper) asked rhetorically, "What Is He Afraid Of?" Above the headline, two red bullet points gave background to the story: "Anwar refuses to give blood sample for DNA test" and "Possibility of bringing in foreign medical experts to conduct tests." Underneath, in large letters, was a quote from Datuk Seri Syed Hamid Albar, Home Minister: "If he's searching for the truth, he can get it very easily. Just give a blood sample for DNA tests. . . . Under our laws, we cannot force a person to give a blood sample." On an inside page, the main news story was reported under another headline, also a quotation from the Home Minister: "Give blood sample for the sake of truth." Other newspapers in Malaysia ran this story with the same prominence.

These headlines came at a climactic moment in a long-running and increasingly surreal saga in Malaysian politics, in which several news stories seemed somehow to converge on a DNA analysis of the blood of Datuk Seri Anwar Ibrahim, the de facto leader of the main opposition party, Parti Keadilan Rakyat (PKR, People's Justice Party), and longtime thorn in the government's side. The many bizarre turns in this sequence of events almost defy summary, but for someone engaged at the time in research on the interface between biomedical understandings of blood and its wider symbolic resonances in Malaysia, the moment seemed almost too extraordinary to be believed. How had Anwar's blood come to be claimed by the government as an icon of truth in a tumultuous political showdown?[1]

General elections in March 2008 had resulted in very significant gains for the opposition parties. For the first time since 1969, the ruling alliance of government parties (Barisan Nasional) headed by UMNO had lost its two-thirds majority in Parliament—but not its overall majority—and the opposition parties had won a number of key states. A background of increasing dissatisfaction among voters, particularly over what was perceived as widespread corruption in government, and stories of scandals implicating leading politicians had led to this result. It was conjectured by some that the decades of UMNO rule might be nearing an end. In the weeks and months following the election, Anwar stepped up an increasingly direct attack on a faltering government, and particularly on the reputation of Deputy Prime Minister Datuk Seri Najib Tun Razak. This hinged on allegations about the latter's embroilment in the murder of a Mongolian translator, Altantuya Shaariibuu, by means of C4 explosives, which had allegedly been committed to cover up a sex and corruption scandal involving prominent government figures. The case was one of several high-profile ones then being tried in the Malaysian courts.

After the election, Anwar repeatedly boasted that, by the following September, sufficient MPs from parties in the ruling Barisan Nasional (particularly from the states of East Malaysia, Sabah and Sarawak) would achieve a majority, and the government would fall. It was perhaps not surprising to observers familiar with Malaysian politics that the government would respond to such direct provocation. On June 29, in a bizarre reprise of events ten years before, under the Mahathir government, when Anwar had been sacked as Deputy Prime Minister and arrested and jailed for sodomy, the story broke in the Malaysian press that one of Anwar's aides, Mohd Saiful Bukhari, had lodged a report with the police alleging sodomy by the PKR leader.[2] On the same day, amid claims that he had received death threats, Anwar took refuge in the Turkish embassy. He emerged from there on July 1 after assurances for his personal safety had been given by the Home Minister and the Deputy Prime Minister. On the same day, Mohd Saiful was exposed in photographs released by Parti Keadilan Rakyat as having links to the office of the Deputy Prime Minister. According to a report in *The Star*, at a press conference on July 3, Anwar "declared that evidence linking deputy Prime Minister Najib to the murdered Mongolian translator will be released in the coming days." Describing the Altantuya case as "like a series in a Bollywood drama," he also accused the police of suppressing evidence and questioned "why there was a sudden switching of the judge fixed to hear the case."[3]

Following his arrest on July 16, Anwar was taken to the main hospital in Kuala Lumpur, where, according to accounts in the Malaysian media, he was medically examined but refused to give a blood sample for DNA testing, fearing that it might be tampered with. In a statement alleging that he had been stripped naked during this examination, which was denied by the director of the hospital, Datuk Dr. Zaininah Mohd Zain, Anwar was reported as saying,

> "They measured me and examined me, front and back," ... when meeting PKR members at party headquarters in Petaling Jaya later yesterday.
>
> He said the police should not ask for his DNA sample again as they had taken his blood samples many times when he was in prison for six years.
>
> "I had my blood tested many times for sugar level, cholesterol. But now they say those were old DNA samples," he added.[4]

In the heightened atmosphere of the time, and amid increasingly vitriolic accusations leveled in all directions, the role of Anwar's blood in this story was just one of many remarkable subthemes. For not only were his previous blood samples presumably available to the police but, as at least some bloggers commented, if DNA was at issue, blood was not required. A simple mouth swab, for example, might have been easier to acquire. So, what was it about blood, as distinct from, say, saliva or hair, that had the capacity to reveal the truth? Or was it perhaps not just the blood but also the idea of "the sample" and its scientific testing, possibly verified by "foreign medical experts," that would supply the desired authenticity for this rather questionable evidence?[5]

These reports came at an extraordinary juncture in Malaysian public life, when the political moment and my research appeared to converge in a quite unanticipated way. A contested blood sample from the leader of the opposition alliance was claimed by some as having the capacity to reveal the truth about his character. Significantly perhaps, what exactly the blood sample was supposed to show in this case was not explicitly spelled out in the reports in the Malaysian press. One might surmise that the authorities were either hoping to match samples produced by Anwar's political aide or perhaps were seeking a positive HIV test (which would not require DNA). This, however, was left implicit, and thus presumably all the more open to different interpretations that might cast aspersions on his character.

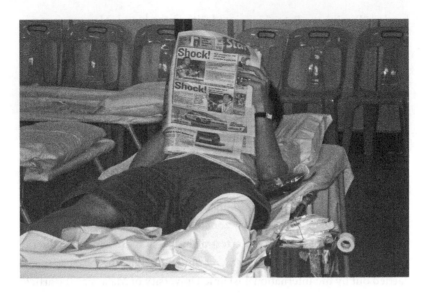

A blood donor reads of the tumultuous events of 2008 in *The Star*.

A few months prior to these events, it was reported in the press that Prime Minister Abdullah Badawi, campaigning in Penang some weeks before the elections, had expounded on the spirit of inclusiveness and harmony characterizing Malaysia: "I am a Malay but I am prime minister of all races—that was Prime Minister Datuk Seri Abdullah Ahmad Badawi's message to the people," began *The Star*'s report.[6] And he cited his long-term friendships with Chinese and Indian school friends as evidence of these attitudes. The article noted that the Prime Minister also spoke of his duty "as a Muslim . . . to be 'honest and fair' to everyone regardless of their race or religion." At the elections, however, Penang was one of five states gained by the opposition alliance. And while informal conversations with almost everyone I encountered immediately before the elections—including hospital workers, intellectuals, taxi drivers, hairdressers, activists, and private teachers—suggested that this might happen, the scale of the victory took most by surprise.

During the election campaign, there was much comment on the importance of familial connections between many of Malaysia's leading political figures, especially a new younger generation of politicians. An article headed "Passing the Baton" suggested, "It's in the blood. Many sons of political fathers are following the campaign trails."[7] Interestingly, however, the blood in question apparently combined both "nature" and "nurture." The article began, "Thanks to nature and nurture, politics runs in their blood. It comes as no surprise that many children of political parents follow in their footsteps, especially if they have grown up in a political environment." But the familial register was not the only mode in which blood could seep into political matters. We have seen in chapters 1 and 2 the way in which a loose set of associations between attributes or behavior, religion, ethnicity, and what is locally termed "race" suffuses life in Malaysia and in some circumstances can encompass blood and organ donation or other matters. Exemplifying this tendency, in February 2008, shortly after street demonstrations in Kuala Lumpur following the arrest of Indian activists, an article in *The Star* reported on "an election survey," commissioned by the newspaper and carried out by the International Islamic University of Malaysia. The article began, "All three major races in the country are against demonstrations and illegal gatherings in Kuala Lumpur." It was illustrated with a bar chart showing separately the "views on street demonstrations in KL" for Malays, Chinese, and Indians, and also giving the total for all these groups. The main part of the article contained a detailed analysis of the figures over many paragraphs. I cite just one here: "Among the three races, the Indians made up the highest number of people who 'agree' with the demonstrations—at 16%. Three percent of Indians chose 'fully agree,' while 1% had no response."[8] One specter that lurks behind such discourse, and which is relevant to the timing of this article during the election campaign, is the memory of the riots between Malays and Chinese in Kuala Lumpur that broke out on May 13, 1969, a few days after the only other election in which the governing Alliance Party failed to get a two-thirds majority.

The events of 1969, which according to some commentators were not spontaneous but a planned move against Prime Minister Tunku Abdul Rahman, by members of his own party, mark a kind of caesura and a defining moment in the history of Malaysia. The official tally of 196 killed in these events is at wide variance with other sources which suggest that between 800 and 1,000 people lost their lives. As well as a spate of detentions of opposition politicians under the notorious ISA (Internal Security Act), the declaration of a state of emergency, and the formation of a National

Operations Council with the suspension of Parliament for nearly two years, these events led to a realignment in Malaysian politics, including in 1973 the formation of a new ruling coalition, the Barisan Nasional (Kua 2007; Means 1999, 21–25).

On May 11, 2008, *The Star* marked the thirty-ninth anniversary of the riots with a thoughtful two-page discussion piece on which I draw here, titled "Truth and Reconciliation," by journalist Martin Vengadesan. Noting the lack of victory celebrations and the palpable air of tension in Malaysian cities in the few days following the elections of March 2008, this article drew comparisons between 1969 and 2008 and compiled the views of various witnesses to and social commentators on the earlier events. Dr. Kua Kia Soong, author of *May 13: Declassified Documents on the Malaysian Riots of 1969* (2007) and director of the Malaysian human rights organization SUARAM, who was himself detained under the ISA in the 1980s, was quoted as stating,

> May 13 is part of our history and is consistently trotted out by politicians who want to play the racial card, to show us what will happen if the privileges of the ruling class are threatened. We need to have a process of truth and reconciliation.[9]

Although many politicians in Malaysia have for decades relied on the events of 1969 and promulgated an essentialist vision of the differences between Malay, Chinese, and Indian Malaysians, the election results of 2008 seemed to confound this view. They suggested that the expected connections between "race" and political alignments could also be severed, and the implications of this were widely commented upon. It would take another ten years, however, until the general elections of May 2018, in which the ruling Barisan Nasional lost its majority for the first time, for the assumed connections between ethnicity and party allegiance to be decisively upturned. In view of the prevailing discourse that I have described here, it was perhaps not surprising that conversations with blood donors or with staff who worked in the blood banks and medical pathology labs sometimes revealed stereotyped views about Malays or Chinese. But the people I encountered in these locations also upturned such expectations—as we will see in the chapters that follow.

That the results of the general election of March 8 were broadly unexpected was indicated by the tone of media reports as well as by subsequent events. In a memorable front-page headline on March 9, *The Star* called the results a "Political Tsunami"—a metaphor that was widely echoed. Expectations about voting patterns among different groups, built up over the fifty years since independence, were upset. While the ruling Barisan Nasional headed by UMNO had not been brought down, it had lost its two-thirds majority, the guarantor of being able to make changes to the constitution. For the first time in many years, it seemed conceivable that the status quo might change, and the future of the Barisan Nasional, and of UMNO, looked considerably less secure.

In spite of the consistent calls on their loyalties from the ruling parties, it was clear that many voters—particularly, urban Malay, Indian, and Chinese Malaysians in Penang and Kuala Lumpur—had deserted their historical ethnic political allegiances to parties of the Barisan Nasional, that is to UMNO (the United Malays National Organisation), the MIC (Malaysian Indian Congress), and the MCA (the Malaysian Chinese Association), and instead voted for a coalition of opposition parties headed by Anwar Ibrahim. Partly because the opposition alliance included the Islamic PAS (Parti se Islam Malaysia), as well as more straightforwardly centrist and left-wing parties (including some with ethnic ties), its success relied on some voters giving their support to parties and leaders that crossed ethnic lines and upset past voting patterns. After the elections it was widely agreed that the opposition had also made far better use of new communication technologies (including blogging and cell phones) and that its supporters included many younger voters.[10]

For some days and weeks after the election, the atmosphere was heady; people everywhere discussed the results and the possible consequences for the government. It was clear that Prime Minister Abdullah Ahmad Badawi's position was shaky, and the two long-term political opponents, Deputy Prime Minister Najib Tun Razak and Anwar Ibrahim, lined up for what seemed an increasingly fateful confrontation. When, in a calculated move, on May 19 the former Prime Minister of more than twenty years, Tun Dr. Mahathir Mohamad, resigned his membership of UMNO and called on others to do the same, the Prime Minister seemed unlikely to survive for long. A handover to Najib was widely predicted to take place later in the year, and did so in 2009.

These events generated widespread excitement and were talked about in many contexts with animation and interest. In the hospital clinical pathology labs and blood banks the atmosphere was generally quiet and subdued—these were hardly political hotbeds. But a few of the medical lab technologists talked about political meetings they had attended before the election and, like the majority of Penangites, most seemed likely to support the opposition parties. Immediately following the election, I spent some time in the dialysis unit of one of the hospitals. Patients there attended regularly for two or three sessions a week lasting several hours; some had gotten to know each other well over many years and had requested customary places for dialysis treatment near these friends. I was impressed in particular by a double row of male patients in facing reclining chairs at the center of the unit, who spent their time talking politics while consuming snacks in a manner that reminded me of the men in village coffee shops on the Malaysian island of Langkawi I had known in the early 1980s.

When the political atmosphere intensified in July 2008, there was a sense that this escalation had been overdetermined. But the centrality of the contested evidence of a blood sample to these political events, and the link between the sample and Anwar's moral status was unexpected.[11] The truth that would emerge, however, was at the time left quite unspecified in these reports—it is not at all clear what could be ascertained through the sample or the tests to which it might be subjected. In the context of widespread incredulity, it seemed that the government sought to lend legitimacy to Anwar's arrest through scientific tests. Or perhaps what was being sought was a vivid reminder to opponents of the government of Anwar's previous imprisonment under the same charge and the power of the state that could be brought to bear on the political opposition.

Anwar Ibrahim's reported resistance to supplying the required blood sample was equally telling. Apparently supposed to reveal whether he had had sex with one of his aides—in other words his moral status—the sample's power lay in its capacity to verify a matter that debatably was only knowable by the two protagonists. One might conclude that the purpose of obtaining this sample had deliberately been left unclear to encourage different kinds of speculation about his moral probity. The potential instability of the meanings of this particular blood sample inhered in layers of history—

not just a general history of the manner in which Malaysian politics had been conducted over several decades, to which I have alluded here, but also a very particular history relating to Anwar's previous arrest and imprisonment (and subsequent release) on the very same charge under the Mahathir government (see Trowell 2015, 44–58). While for the government it might be obvious that Anwar's moral corruption would emerge in unanswerable terms from the analysis of a sample, for a substantial part of the Malaysian public, the story as presented seemed to lack credibility. The blood sample, in other words, might reveal truths quite unintended by the government.

These newspaper reports convey the events and general atmosphere of Malaysia in 2008. They give a sense of the social, political, and moral issues that were current in public discourse and that imbued ordinary people's lives. The accounts highlight how easily discourses about blood at this particular juncture in Malaysia could move between its literal qualities, including medical meanings, and more metaphorical understandings. Rather than clarifying Anwar's moral status, what emerged from this sample was the excess of meanings pertaining to blood. The polyvalent meanings of blood itself, and the resonances between its material, medical, and moral connotations, readily become self-evident as they flow between the multiple fields and discourses in which blood participates. The possibilities that exist for inserting blood or organ donation into discourses that are heavily politically inflected are suggestive of the capacity these bodily materials have for metaphorical extension. They indicate both the importance of excluding such resonances of blood from work in the labs through boundary work and the difficulties of so doing.

As I was observing one of the senior staff, Emily, whom I had known since early in my research in 2008, instructing a trainee in medical lab technology in 2012, she told me that, when she was examining slides for anomalies, she tried not to think about the sources of samples in patients. To underline her point, she related how the trainee who was working beside her had recently attended a bone marrow aspiration and had become nauseated because the process was clearly painful for the patient.

> So, the trainee has to learn to distinguish. Most trainees don't have a problem—but sometimes—bone marrow aspiration—[trainees] turn green. The trainees are like patients—when draw blood, sometimes turn green. For us it's our job—we learn to distinguish. When [they] see blood coming out from the body it's different.

Such processes of separation are intrinsic to the work of the lab, but it is also clear from the different ways that trainees engage with their learning that it is often the connections between tasks in the lab and the lives of patients that animate their interest. Making and unmaking such separations are thus always ambivalent and unstable processes that proceed simultaneously (see Singleton 1998, 97). Learning the skills necessary for work in the clinical pathology labs requires training and concentration, and without these skills, in the view of senior staff, lab work would not be possible. A central aspect of this work is the analysis of patient samples.

During the months I spent in the clinical pathology labs and blood banks, I had many occasions to observe trainees learning the procedures that were carried out in different departments. Sometimes I would happen upon them looking rather bored as they laboriously and meticulously copied out printed sheets of standard operating procedures for a particular task.

This seemed to be their least favorite way of learning, and I wondered how much they really learned about how to do things through this method. At other times, I came across one of the more senior medical lab technologists demonstrating a procedure, such as how to take blood from a donor, or how to enter required information about the donor into the blood bank information system and donor record book, directly to the trainees. It was at these points that trainees immediately became much more attentive and alert, as standard operating procedures were brought to life. Often the medical lab technologist would ask questions at the time or later to make sure trainees had understood properly, and sometimes, as I describe more fully in chapter 4, these conversations would divert to discussions about matters of more general interest, such as marriage or finances. Once they had spent a little time in any of the departments, trainees were shown how to do some tasks themselves, which were carried out independently under supervision from the staff stationed there. And at these moments it became apparent that they were much more concentrated on and engaged with what they were doing.

• • •

This chapter focuses on the work carried out in the clinical pathology labs and blood banks. Most of this work is highly technical, and it comes in the form of many small, intricate tasks. There are literally hundreds of diagnostic tests that labs may be equipped to do in their different departments on blood, sputum, urine, stool, or other samples. And diagnostic testing is only one part of the work of the labs. The medical lab technologists (MLTS), phlebotomists, and lab technicians are also responsible for taking blood from blood donors, screening blood, separating and preparing blood as components, storing and refrigerating components, managing blood bank supplies, and cross-matching blood for transfusion with that of patients. The lab staff also take blood from hospital inpatients and outpatients before testing it, and they make sure the results of the diagnostic tests they carry out in the different departments of the lab are accurately recorded and speedily transmitted back to wards and outpatient clinics. A full description of the hundreds of tasks involved in this work would take more space than is available here. Instead, I highlight some of the ways that the social engagement of lab staff penetrates even the most technical aspects of their work.

In her suggestive analysis of the role of the laboratory in the UK cervical cancer screening program, Vicky Singleton (1998) shows how variations in the way lab work is carried out, and divergences from set protocols, create instabilities in the constituent processes of lab work. Rather than the many component processes adhering to their set roles in order for the program to achieve its aims—as would be suggested by actor-network theory— she argues that cervical cells, "samples, report cards, sample takers and women assume a multiplicity of identities through laboratory discourse and practice, some of which do not readily fit into the CSP [Cervical Screening Programme] as defined by the government and as publicly represented" (1998, 92). The resulting instabilities, however, instead of contributing to the instability of the screening program itself or being a threat to laboratory practice, are accommodated within the work of the lab and in fact contribute to the accommodation of other instabilities and ambivalences in components of the program outside the lab: "Laboratory discourse suggests that the ability of the laboratory to detect precancerous cytological changes depends on its ability to accommodate instability and ambiguity" (1998, 103). Far from being a threat or source of conflict to the work of the lab or the screening program as a whole, Singleton suggests that the accommodation of instability at the level of laboratory practice actually allows stability at the level of the CSP to be maintained. Her conclusion, that instability and ambivalence should be seen as a necessary part of this kind of diagnostic lab work, is highly relevant for the lab work I describe here, in which we can trace similar instabilities and uncertainties.

Many of the processes that I observed began with the extraction of bodily fluids or tissue from patients or donors. These samples were then examined or analyzed before results were recorded and entered into the information systems of the lab; the results were then transmitted to doctors or nurses. The processes of extraction, analysis, storage, disposal, and data recording are at the heart of what goes on in the labs. This involves taking something internal to the human body and transforming it into a detached object of scientific analysis and then into recorded information. This of course cannot happen without social engagement, and it is this that concerns me here. Examining a few of the many hundreds of work processes carried out in the labs and blood banks, I attend to the forms of social relations that occur—beginning with the interactions between medical lab technologists and blood donors or patients (such as those I described in chapter 1), but also encompassing those between working colleagues and between the staff of the labs and the samples they analyze, as well as those between the staff and the equipment they use. My questions concern these engagements: if the blood donors who come to give blood are imbued with social and moral qualities, as we saw from newspaper accounts and in chapter 1, is this in any sense also true of blood products stored in triple packs under refrigeration, or of the blood samples in test tubes that are screened, or of those taken from patients to test for particular diseases? How is the transition from bodies to samples, or from social relations to an object of analysis, effected? What kinds of "technologies of detachment"[1] or processes of "purification" (Latour 1993) does this involve? And what can these processes tell us about blood as a particular kind of unstable substance or about the social relations initiated here? Finally, is there anything that is particularly Malaysian in the way this work is carried out or in the social engagements that I describe? Attempting to answer these questions is not the task of this chapter alone but also of the one that follows, in which I focus more exclusively on the lives of people who work in the labs and the relations they have with their colleagues.

Part of my argument here is that the transformation of blood from bodily substance into laboratory object apparently involves divesting it of the social qualities it carries. This can be seen as one effect of the particular kind of work that goes on in the clinical pathology labs. But I also suggest that, partly because of its polysemic meanings and qualities and its derivation from human bodies, this divestment is at best unstable. The detachment of the personal or moral attributes of blood remains provisional, and we can also observe how such qualities may be reattributed or newly attributed through the engagements of social actors in the labs. Analogous to the cervical screening lab discussed by Singleton, here it is blood packs and samples that are ambivalent and unstable objects. Rather than undermining the work of the lab, however, we see how the multiple engagement of lab staff, and their attempts to "rehumanize" their workspaces and tasks, actually secures their continued interest in routine work and enhances the quality of lab results. Thus, although my opening vignette suggested that learning detachment was at the heart of the on-the-job experience that trainees gain, we will see that high-quality work also rests on imaginative human engagement with samples and patients. We also see how, through these processes, ethics and politics are enfolded within the very processes of the labs (see Mol and Berg 1998, 8). And this underlines the argument made in the introduction to this book—not only that blood is itself a "multiple" object but that this multiplicity extends from blood donation (see chapter 1) to laboratory processes and to the many biomedical sites in which blood participates (Berg and Mol 1998). In order to begin to trace how this multiplicity is enacted in the lab, I first describe how blood is extracted from patients and then follow some of the pathways along which it travels.

Taking Blood from Patients

My field notes from research in 2008 and from subsequent visits are full of descriptions of "blood-taking events"—some of these extremely brief, some longer and fuller—but at the time none of them seemed quite satisfactory or complete. Each attempt at description captured part but not all of the minute actions and interactions that occurred in just a few minutes. Encounters between patients and MLTs varied, as did the practices of individual MLTs, and since they worked with different partners, the nature of these working relationships also marked how they carried out these tasks and their engagements with patients. But with hindsight, the incompleteness registered in my notes is suggestive. Over many months, I watched MLTs take blood from patients probably hundreds of times. The procedures were so quick and so routinized that they were difficult to absorb properly, and often I seemed to miss some crucial part of what had happened. Within a few minutes it was all over.

Blood samples were taken by medical lab technologists or phlebotomists from inpatients in their beds on the hospital wards, from outpatients at the outpatient section of the clinical pathology labs, and for screening purposes from blood donors who came either to the blood bank or to external blood donation drives (as described in chapter 1). In all cases there was a standard procedure to be followed, but in actuality there were a surprising number of very minor variations, depending partly on who was taking the blood. The differences between depictions in my notes taken on different days are thus in themselves revealing.

In many cases, the medical lab technologist hardly engaged with patients at all beyond asking their names. And so, the taking of blood was often what one might call a "barely social" encounter. From the MLTs' point of view, it did not seem that chatting to or engaging with patients was required or even expected. This contrasted with the usually more sociable behavior of nurses toward patients. But it was also clear that different patients had different expectations, and most of them were responsive when the MLTs did talk to them while taking a blood sample. Some patients would recognize a medical lab technologist from a previous encounter. The patient might have been in the hospital for some time or had perhaps been in before, and would strike up a conversation or would voice a preference for which medical lab technologist should take their blood (generally opting for the senior one, or the one whom they knew had taken blood before least painfully). Some of the MLTs were distinctly more chatty than others and more likely to engage with patients when they were taking their blood. In a few cases, the medical lab technologists showed that they knew quite a lot about a particular patient, their illness, and their family life. Sometimes they checked on a patient's progress—either by asking the nurses on the ward before leaving or by checking the hospital information system later from the lab computers. Quite often, particular patients whom they had seen on the wards were discussed later among the MLTs in the labs. One morning, an elderly patient whose blood had been taken the previous day died on the ward. I was surprised at how much the MLTs knew about him—as my field notes indicated:

> Ai Wen and Min Hui tell me about an 88-year-old patient—they think perhaps from the UK—who has just died on Surgical 1—this must be the reason for the alarms when we were up in the ward. Ai Wen says this is the rhesus negative patient that she had to get blood for yesterday. He had a stroke and multiple fractures. Had been living in a hotel for the last 12 years, had no family. Was brought in by a friend. I ask Min Hui whether she talked to him—she says only a bit. Bunga gets a urine test request form for the same patient. Min Hui says to ask them to cancel the charges as the test won't be run now. Eng Swee wipes her eyes— and I'm not sure whether this is because she is upset or not. But in any case, they are obviously upset. In the blood bank there is a form from [name of another hospital] saying 1 unit of O negative "borrowed from XXX." "To return 2 units O type whole blood." Ai Wen says this was used yesterday—"I think [he had] internal bleeding."

In the previous chapter, I described some of the different kinds of people and social dispositions found among the lab staff. It was from their encounters with patients that I first learned how some viewed their job rather like an alternative to nursing, while others particularly valued the peace and quiet of the labs—its apparent detachment from intense social engagement. Because of the nature of their work, more sociable exchanges with patients or knowledge about their backgrounds were often mixed up with various bits of medical information.

There were differences too between the MLTs in how they observed hygiene procedures when they took blood. Some always wore latex gloves on both hands when they took blood; others sometimes did, or usually wore gloves on one hand but not both. Some always washed their hands before leaving each ward. Sometimes this was done after taking blood from a particular patient. The variations were partly idiosyncratic, and the MLTs were not necessarily consistent in when and how they used latex gloves or washed their hands. Occasionally, it was obvious that they were being particularly careful—disposing of a tourniquet they had tied around a patient's arm as well as their gloves, and washing their hands after taking blood from a particular patient. Usually, this was a patient whose blood was being tested for HIV. And once again there might be discussion back in the labs that revealed how different kinds of understanding could become entangled with the process of getting lab results: Was the patient Indonesian? Did he have bruising or other marks on his skin? Was he good-looking? Did he seem young? These kinds of questions or comments suggested that HIV status went together with other physical, personal, or moral attributes. Such comments circulated in the lab at the same time as the patient's blood sample in a Vacutainer, with a red sticker affixed to indicate that special caution should be observed. If the patient in question was female, it seemed to be assumed that she had been infected by her husband. The questions of staff then were more likely to concern her familial status and comments to indicate that they felt sorry for her. These conversations recall Naomi Pfeffer and Sophie Laws's discussion of how the apparent insignificance of blood testing events in the UK masks a more complex reality in which blood tests "can also provide incriminating information about people as moral agents" (2006, 3015).

Lab staff were under pressure to observe hygiene protocols when taking blood from patients and handling their samples. From the point of view of hospital management, this was partly a matter of conforming to the standards required for external accreditation, which might be verified by inspection visits or sometimes commented on by patients. For staff, this was also about ensuring their own safety, and they certainly took care not to compromise this. But practices could vary in ways that made the implications of seemingly standard safety precautions less clear than they might appear. When an MLT had taken blood from a patient on the ward, she would pass the hypodermic syringe with the sharp attached to her partner. The partner would insert the needle into the caps of the required sample tubes, filling each to the required level, before removing the sharp and attached hypodermic and disposing of them. In one hospital the first MLT would always take care to cap the needle before passing it pointed upward to her partner, and this was regarded as the safest way to perform this task. This seemed to make sense until I observed how, in another hospital, the same basic practices were observed and needles were also always passed pointed upward, but this time uncapped. When I asked about this, I was told that studies had revealed that more accidents were likely to occur by trying to cap used needles than by passing them uncapped.[2] The wearing of latex gloves too could have unexpected implications. One MLT who was very concerned about hygiene often commented that wearing gloves encouraged a kind of complacency, so that staff would complete several tasks wearing the same gloves when in fact their hands were no longer clean. He himself preferred to wear gloves less and wash his hands more.

Although hygiene practices often struck me as one of the more variable features of the way in which blood was taken from patients, MLTs themselves talked of the ways skill, experience, and luck entered into their work. As I spent more time with them, I became accustomed to seeing how carefully they inserted the needle into the patient's vein. Sometimes it took repeated efforts to succeed in taking blood. It might be hard to find a suitable vein in the arm—particularly if patients were elderly or obese—and it was important to get the angle of insertion right. The MLTs explained to me how a steeper angle of the syringe to the vein increased the draw. It was easier to take blood from a patient lying on a flat bed than if the patient was sitting or the bed was raised, because the arm was already at an angle, and the syringe had to be raised higher. Narrow veins could be fragile; a vein might collapse after the needle was inserted, and then a different vein would have to be chosen—perhaps from the back of the hand, where narrower veins required smaller needles.

When two MLTs were working together on the wards, they sometimes switched roles when one partner was having difficulties finding a suitable vein. Or if they were working in the outpatient section, it was not uncommon to call in a more experienced colleague to help. Some colleagues were seen as particularly skilled in phlebotomy, but the MLTs said that this was also partly a matter of luck. One told me it was "mainly experience—80 percent experience, 20 percent luck." She then told me about one of the junior colleagues, a phlebotomist who was very good even though she was less experienced: she had a "special technique of slightly turning the needle when it's in—just her—never seen anyone else do it." Some vividly recalled how scared they had been the first time they had had to take blood. One told me, "My hands were shaking. I felt the pain as if I was the patient. The first three or four months like that." Another said, "My hands were cold." And I witnessed this myself when I saw one young man being trained as a phlebotomist. Over a few weeks, he accompanied different pairs of MLTs as they went around the wards. He learned through a combination of instruction and being encouraged to take blood himself under supervision. In this case, his preference for watching rather than doing was clear, and provoked quite a lot of teasing from the MLTs training him. When he graduated to taking blood himself, they were careful to comment on his technique only after they left the wards. Then they would remind him of the importance of getting the angle of the syringe right or correct his use of alcohol swabs, telling him it was better not to use the same swab and rub many times but instead to use two swabs. They also said to check the needle to see if an air bubble had entered the syringe. But they told me that he was already skilled—it was "just a matter of experience." On another day, the trainee had a problem taking blood when there was an air bubble in the syringe. Later the MLT training him said to me that after they left the ward she had told him there were three possible reasons for this: either the needle didn't go deep enough so that air entered, or the needle was not screwed on tight enough, or he hadn't pushed the plunger all the way down first so there was air in the syringe before. She herself didn't know which was the case: "I told him he has to find out for himself."

When I asked MLTs to talk me through what was involved in taking blood, I was interested to hear the differences between them. Their animated descriptions also showed that they were very aware of the small discrepancies in preferred techniques of colleagues as well as between the veins of patients that might make taking blood difficult. There were some among the MLTs who took special pride in being able to take blood without causing the patients pain. One was pointed out to me by several of his colleagues as unusual in being able to take blood from himself. This was obviously regarded as something of a feat, made possible, they said, by his very long fingers. And so, personal preferences and idiosyncrasies, skill, experience, and a little luck, as well as different degrees of social engagement with patients, entered into this single routine procedure of the lab. Significantly, we have seen how many experienced staff members recalled their fears of taking blood from early in their careers when, like the trainee in my opening vignette, they had not yet learned the separations necessary for lab work. The vividness with which such memories were recounted is suggestive of the hard work intrinsic to making such separations and the instabilities of blood itself as a purified object.

Samples, Testing, and Screening

Different labs had differently organized information systems for data entry and recording. But in all cases, the samples were logged in—and this might be done by a receptionist or someone else in the lab responsible for data entry. Normally, most of the information for patients had already been entered by registration staff and nurses on the wards or at outpatient clinics.

When I asked one of the lab managers for a list of the tests performed in the lab, he kindly printed one off for me—it covered thirty-one A4 pages with perhaps an average of twenty-five tests on each. Some of these came in groups or "packages" for particular types of patients (those being tested for heart disease or diabetes, for example), or a category of corporate insurance coverage, which came with standard routine tests. Some were performed for many patients each day; some were requested relatively rarely. Different kinds of tests were automated to different degrees, and this partly depended on the lab size and level of equipment. For example, the standard tests in blood chemistry and immunology were very highly automated, with batches of Vacutainers arranged in racks to pass through a sophisticated blood analyzer. Several hundred analyses of blood chemistry and immunology, testing levels of blood sugar, cholesterol, different hormones, lipids, proteins, or enzymes, the presence or absence of drugs or of specific cancer markers, as well as the screening of donated blood or that of patients for syphilis, hepatitis A, B, and C antibodies, hepatitis C virus (HCV), and HIV could be performed in a few hours. But some immunological and other tests—such as those for dengue fever, lupus, and lactose intolerance, or further confirmatory tests for HIV—were performed individually or in very small numbers by MLTs, using kits that required careful and precise measurement. On a few occasions I followed senior members of staff when they conducted less routine procedures, such as preparation of a sample for a fertility procedure such as IUI (intrauterine insemination) or genetic testing of tissue for breast cancer.

The blood counts for hemoglobin and different white and red cells, as well as platelets in the blood and ESR (erithrocyte sedimentation rate), that were performed in the hematology departments were also performed in batches mechanically. But when the analyzer showed abnormal results, further testing was conducted by staining and fixing a slide, which was then examined by the MLT under a microscope. Standard operating procedures were subject to change as new machinery or diagnostic tools became available. Blood grouping was done manually in the labs I observed, but when I visited one lab after an absence of some months, a new machine had been acquired for blood grouping and cross-matching. Tests in the urinalysis and bacteriology departments required more manual intervention, and some of the analysis also involved visual examination—for example to report on the color or cloudiness of urine, or checking cultures of bacterial growth in petri dishes. Some tests were newly introduced while I was in the labs, which sometimes coincided with the introduction of new equipment or the arrival of a new consultant at the hospital who specialized in a particular branch of medicine.

Several of the older staff in the lab spontaneously spoke of how the work of the labs had been altered during their time there by increasing technologization. Some could remember when almost all the tests were done manually and far fewer tests were carried out in the labs—many were sent out. But it was clear from the work preferences of MLTs that increasing automation was not necessarily seen as a good thing. Reducing their own intervention also made the work much more routinized. One MLT

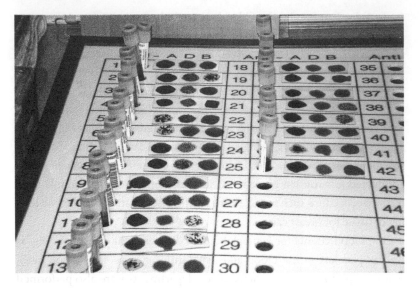

Slides are arranged on a lab bench for blood grouping (manual method).

commented specifically that it was because of the degree of mechanization that he thought the work was more suited to women than men. We saw in chapter 2 that the majority of those who work in the labs are women. The kinds of emotional investments made in the work processes as well as the social relations between colleagues can thus be seen as gendered labor. Several other MLTs told me that they preferred working in the parts of the lab that were less automated, such as microbiology—even though, because of the risks of infection, one might have expected growing bacterial cultures from stool, sputum, or other samples to be a less favored work task. It was clear that, for most MLTs, the aspects of the work which gave satisfaction were those that involved making their own judgments, especially when these led to a tricky or unexpected diagnosis. In this sense, much like the trainees described in the opening section to this chapter, who became animated when they directly engaged in lab work, the senior staff preferred it when the work was less highly automated and when their own skilled interventions, based on experience and knowledge, were integral to achieving results.

When a complex and expensive piece of new technology for blood grouping and cross-matching, which also recorded the data digitally, was introduced in one lab, the staff's comments indicated that they were skep-

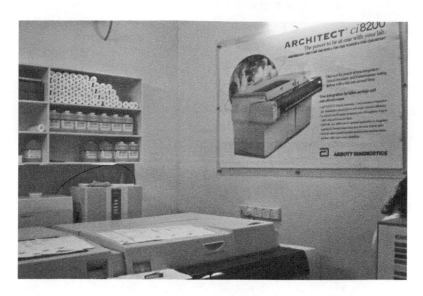

The blood analyzer is one high-tech tool in the lab.

tical about how much time it saved. This was partly because it took time to get results and partly because the analyzer seemed to be very sensitive and liable to stop working if the chemical reagents used were not at exactly the right levels. While I looked on over a short period one morning, the analyzer's alarm went off several times to indicate that it had run out of reagent. When one of the MLTs came to check, she said it was because the bar code on the reagent had not been aligned properly with the sensor. The new machine could take up to forty samples and ascertain blood groups of these in thirty minutes, and this included reverse grouping to confirm the results. But one experienced member of staff told me that the old method of determining blood groups manually (by adding different reagents to three drops of blood on a slide using pipettes, watching the color changes, and recording the results by hand) took "just a few minutes," so if they wanted a quick result, they would still use that. When they operated the manual system, he said, they had only done forward grouping—rather than reverse grouping all samples as a matter of course. Reverse grouping was thus mainly reserved for cross-matching blood for transfusion, where it was imperative that the blood group had been accurately ascertained. But he also acknowledged that with the new technology it was possible for staff to carry out other tasks at the

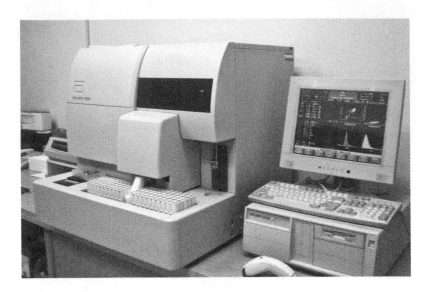

Lab staff rely on technology to do blood work.

same time as blood grouping—for example, looking after blood donors. And I noted that blood grouping had been transferred from the hematology department, where it had been done previously, to the blood bank. The lab manager said that because reverse grouping was now performed on all the samples, and also because the data were no longer recorded manually, the new machine eliminated errors. A further kind of benefit was hinted at when some days later, the CEO of the hospital brought a group of distinguished foreign visitors to tour the lab and pointed out this latest example of the hospital's high-tech equipment, emphasizing its costliness as well as its accuracy. After the visitors left, one of the lab staff commented rather dryly that actually the machine was leased on a system of reagent rental (with regular maintenance and reagents supplied by a medical technology company). This meant that, like most of their larger items of diagnostic technology, it could be returned or exchanged for a newer model when necessary.

The day-to-day maintenance of diagnostic machinery took up a considerable amount of staff time. The more sophisticated and elaborate machines that were heavily used (such as the blood chemistry and immunology analyzers) had daily maintenance programs run early each morning. Depending on how the work rotations of the lab were organized, this could mean some staff having to come on duty an hour or more before colleagues. Machinery was also liable to break down and thus hold up the work of the lab and the reporting of results. Such events generated quite a lot of stress, as doctors and nurses trying to chase results would soon start to phone the labs. When new diagnostic machines were introduced in the labs, some MLTs would be specifically trained in their routine maintenance and became particularly knowledgeable about certain items of technology, but engineers from the medical technology companies were also regular visitors to the labs. On one occasion, when the main blood chemistry and immunology analyzer in one lab had broken down and the two MLTs who were most expert in its operation were absent, there was a certain amount of banter among colleagues, which I recorded in my notes:

> Kamariah is trying to get recalcitrant Architect machine to work. She says "Big brother not there; Mama not there" [referring to the two members of staff with responsibility for the machine]. Shanthi comes to help but clearly it needs lots of coaxing. Kamariah says normally they start running at about 9.15 or 9.30, so by now it's getting a bit late.
>
> Later in the morning, Cheng Poh also says "Architect's mother not there."

Such jokes give a flavor of the working atmosphere of the labs and of the ways in which machines could be lightheartedly anthropomorphized. The humor turned in very Malaysian fashion on the particular kin relations imagined between the machines and their more senior relatives among the lab staff who operated them—a mother and a big brother. Kinship terms were also sometimes used between colleagues. One older male lab technician was always referred to and addressed as "Uncle Sammy" (in English), and one of the MLTs, a married woman in her thirties, was often addressed by putting her name after a Malay kinship prefix, "Mak" or "Kak" (auntie or older sister), depending on who was speaking. The terms were partly ways of marking age or gender when it did not necessarily correlate with seniority of position in the lab. Hierarchical relations could also be humorously exaggerated by terms of address as a way of politely marking, but at the same time dissipating, their connotations—another familiar Malaysian device. Together with gender and age, the terms used in this humorous vein were usually specific to a particular ethnicity. One of the lab managers who was on good terms with his staff was thus sometimes addressed in a friendly joking way by the latter as "Boss" (using the English term) or "Towkay," a term with wide resonance in Malaysia, usually used for a boss or middle-man in more commercial contexts. When I returned to this lab after a period away, I found that two blood analyzers had been named after the lab manager and the most recently appointed junior MLT respectively.

I discuss relations between colleagues more extensively in the following chapter. Here I note how the inanimate equipment of the lab has been drawn into its intimate social world, and this has occurred in a noticeably Malaysian register, one that carries markers of kinship, gender, and ethnicity. This of course raises the question of whether something similar could also happen to samples or to the recorded information derived from them. How possible is it, in other words, to create stable "purified objects" out of material—particularly blood—derived from human bodies?

Labeling

Once they reached the lab, blood and other samples being tested were literally disembodied substances. Blood samples arrived enclosed in sealed test tubes called Vacutainers—a widely used brand of test tubes with many different colored stoppers to indicate which additives are present in the tubes for different kinds of laboratory analysis. Urine and stool samples came in small, transparent, lidded plastic pots. All samples would first be labeled in the wards when MLTs took blood or when urine or other samples were given by patients or in the outpatients section. The labeling system I describe below was the basis for recording test results manually or digitally. Outwardly at least, the rows of test tubes—with their sticky labels affixed, set out on racks on lab benches or ready for the blood chemistry or immunology analyzer, arranged in batches with the same colored stoppers to indicate a particular kind of test—seemed identical in appearance. The labs, as I have noted, used a combination of manual and mechanized procedures but, in the end, results were recorded in the lab information system accessed from their computers. In the most obvious way, samples and recorded information could be seen as objects or as objectified information, divorced from the bodies or persons from which they were derived.

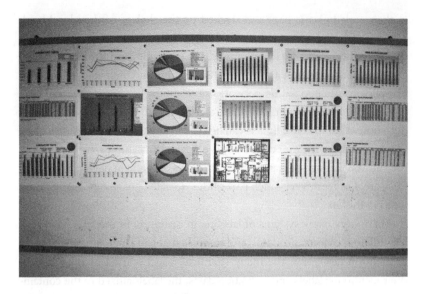

Lab statistics are displayed on a lab wall.

The idea of lab work producing detailed objectified data that were re-corded in information systems was materialized in several ways. Samples labeled with bar codes going through various analyzers in the lab was one. Another was the lab statistics showing the throughput for numbers of tests carried out in each department, which were displayed on notice boards in the form of tables, graphs, or colored pie charts. These demonstrated monthly variation in figures, such as the numbers of tests carried out over one year by a particular department, the proportions of different tests car-ried out by different departments, numbers of units of blood collected (divided into voluntary and replacement donor categories), numbers of re-active screening results for donors (divided into different tests), units of dif-ferent blood components supplied by the blood bank, or the year-over-year increases in numbers of tests carried out by the lab over a period of several years. These were important indicators of the productivity of staff and es-sential tools in discussions with a hospital management that was concerned to improve efficiency and increase profits derived from the lab.

In spite of the detached appearance of such data, for obvious reasons, as they left the lab or even before this, test results or items of recorded in-formation were reconnected to patients. And blood products too, stored in their sealed plastic bags and stacked on the shelves of the blood bank refrigerators, might need to be traced back to their source. Intrigued by the tension between the detached sample, the lab result, and the bag of blood component as objects or as pieces of information, and their source in particular persons situated within networks of relations, I examine the label here as a special kind of material artifact, a component in the "technologies of detachment" of the labs. Labels can be seen as key to the kinds of processes I look at because they mediated between detached samples, or products as they moved through the lab, and their sources of origin in particular people. They are, I suggest, very much part of the "social life of things" (Appadurai 1986) in the lab.

There were many systems of labeling in operation in the lab and countless different objects, products, and samples that had labels affixed to them: to mention just a few, the many chemical reagents used in the lab with their identifying labels and expiration dates; the labels affixed to the containers of patient samples—Vacutainers, petri dishes, small plastic pots; and the labels stuck on bags of donated blood and blood products stored in the blood bank. Here I consider just the labels on patient samples and blood products—beginning with patient samples.

When medical lab technologists collected blood from patients on the wards, they first picked up test request forms from the nurses' stations on each ward. The forms had labels already printed for the sample tubes. The labels gave the patient's hospital number (HN), Identity Card number (IC), name and date of birth (DoB), the kind of test requested, and a bar code. These labels, printed in duplicate, were stuck on the sample tubes and on the form by the lab staff at the time they took blood from the patient. Because the lab bar codes were different from the hospital ones, the MLT would tear off and discard the section with the hospital bar code and affix the part with identification of the patient to the tubes.

Once they were back in the lab, samples were sorted into different trays according to the tubes' different colored caps with their request forms. The receptionist or another member of the lab staff would key the patient's HN into the lab computer, and all the particulars for the patient would then come up on the screen. Registration details for each patient would already have been entered into the hospital information system by registration staff. A receptionist responsible for this process explained to me that if the wrong number was keyed in at the lab this would be immediately obvious. She showed me how when she keyed the hospital number into the lab computer, it generated an access number and bar code for the lab. Next she keyed in the code for each test and the doctor. This information would then come up on every computer in the lab. As she keyed in the hospital number, labels came out of the printer. She would stick the new bar code labels onto the tubes and on the request form from the ward or outpatient clinic. Labels were affixed to each tube and to the patient's request sheet. These labels had the HN, name, sex, DoB, and an access number (bar code number) below the bar code. They also gave the ward and doctor. Each label on each tube for a single patient was the same. One access number was generated for each batch of tests requested by a doctor, which could be for several sample tubes. So it was possible to have several tubes (and more tests) with the same access number. But if the doctor ordered another test later in the day—which could be performed on the same sample as previous tests—this request would generate a new access number and bar code. It was thus possible to have two numbers on one tube. Each bar code number was linked to the access number. The machines in the lab, for example the blood chemistry analyzer, would read the bar code number.

To check a result in the lab, a member of the lab staff keyed in the hospital number and checked the date on which the test had been ordered. Labeled tubes were picked up by staff working in each department. Another member of the lab staff explained how each test result could be approved only on the computer that was linked to the particular machine that ran the test. The results were then printed. Abnormal results would have to be validated—this could be done on any computer in the lab. A lab manager commented that the next step in the development of the information system would be to link the lab computers directly with doctors' requests, so that they wouldn't have to key in tests in the lab. He told me this would take one or two years to be introduced.

Occasionally, a lapse in procedures meant that samples came to the lab unlabeled or wrongly labeled. Because the consequences were potentially very serious, lab staff took great care to avoid such mistakes. When one of the MLTs found a sample tube with no label on it in a bag, she explained to me that there was no way to know whether it was actually from the patient designated on the request form in the same bag. When she phoned the

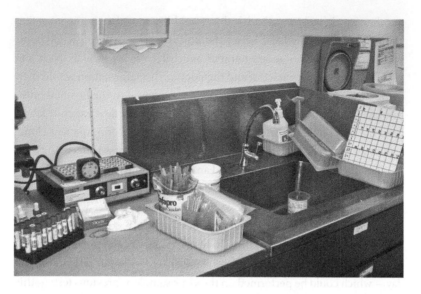

A lab bench includes sample tubes and a sink for blood work.

outpatient section, the phlebotomist who had taken the sample had already gone to lunch. She told me they might have to call the patient back, and both the doctor and the patient would be annoyed. I observed another such mix-up when an MLT phoned the outpatient phlebotomy department about blood that had been wrongly labeled. The phlebotomist hadn't checked the identity of the patient and so would have to take the blood again. The MLT told me that she got very upset about this kind of thing because there was "no need to make the patient suffer twice." On another occasion, I found one of the MLTs working in urinalysis trying to sort out a stool sample that had not been bar-coded. She told me it was "probably because some people don't want to handle a stool sample jar."

It was not just identifying information or the test required that was indicated by labels. One morning while I accompanied one of the MLTs as she was collecting blood from patients on the wards, she showed me a red sticker on the request form to indicate an infectious disease. Sometimes they forget to put a red label on, she said. If the MLT had to use a small needle to take blood she might not be wearing gloves. But they haven't had any serious accidents here, she added. In this instance then, a label communicated special information about precautions to be observed—although all the lab staff were aware that, potentially, any sample might carry risks for the staff who handled it.

Donated blood was also carefully labeled and multiple records were kept of its source. One day I observed as a senior MLT in charge of the blood bank explained the system of labeling donated blood to the new trainees assigned to her. Having taken blood from a voluntary donor, the MLT demonstrated how to print bar code labels for the bags in which blood products were stored. These labels conformed to the International Standard for Blood and Transplant (ISBT). She explained how the forms, blood sample, and blood bags were all bar-coded with donor ID information. Five labels were printed—three for the triple bags used for blood components, one for the form, and one for the Vacutainer containing the patient's blood sample for screening. She showed the trainees the bar code number, M 04 13 08 168043 51(4), which, she explained, designated the source of the blood: M was for Malaysia; 04 indicated Penang; 13 identified the hospital; 08 was the year; 168043 was the donor number; and 51(4) was the computer check digit; the final number in parentheses, she said, was a security number, which changed approximately every twenty donations.[3] But this was not the only record kept of a blood donation. The blood bank's donor record book was completed by hand by the MLT while she was taking blood from a donor. It showed the date, donor number, IC number, age, sex, blood group, hemoglobin (HB) level, address, whether the donor was a volunteer or replacement, and the name of the patient for whom the donor was replacing blood. The MLT explained that this was "in case computer system is down. The donor record book is a backup so that there's no delay getting information."

The MLT showed the trainees how to label each triple bag with a donor number, blood group, bar code, and the different expiration dates for the different components in each bag. She also showed them how to fill in the blood screening record book. Once blood had been taken from donors and blood products had been prepared, it was stored as unscreened blood in a reserve fridge until the screening results were available. The blood bank also kept a separate blood screening results book as a backup in case the computer system was down, in which MLTs recorded by hand the donor number, name, and screening results. Once the screening results were ready, the MLTs would complete the records for each bag that was entered in the donor screening book. Each bag then had a new label affixed to show that it had been screened for HIV, syphilis, and HCV.

When blood was required for transfusion, a request form would arrive in the blood bank from the ward. Sometimes the blood bank did not have adequate stocks of the blood requested and would have to try to source it from outside—usually they tried other local blood banks. But they only used a limited number of these whose screening procedures they trusted and with which they had established exchange relations. If the patient's blood was from a rare group, for example, Rhesus negative, they would sometimes phone potential donors using a list they kept of their own regular donors of Rhesus-negative blood. Assuming the units of requested blood components were available, a sample of the patient's blood first had to be cross-matched with that of the blood components in the blood bank. Once this had been done, the MLT would set out the bags that had been cross-matched in readiness for collection. In addition to the labels that had been affixed at the time the components were prepared, the MLT also attached new colored card labels to requested blood bags ready for the ward—there were different colors for the different components: cryoprecipitate, FFP (fresh frozen plasma), platelets concentrate, and whole blood/packed cells in the different groups: AB positive, A positive, B positive, O positive.

Bags were also logged out in the record book of the blood bank. The blood bank's record book was completed by hand by the blood bank staff, giving the patient's name, hospital number, sex, age, ward, the number of units and blood component required, the blood group of the patient, the "blood matched" (i.e., blood group supplied by the blood bank), bag number, expiration date, confirming compatibility tests, and who had carried these out (i.e., the name of the medical lab technologist). A nurse from the ward would come to the blood bank to collect the required blood with a request form, for example, for two units of fresh frozen plasma. The nurse would check and complete the record in the blood bank record book, filling in the column marked "checked by" with their name and the time and date. Empty used bags and bags of unused blood were brought back and also logged in on the same page as "blood returned" or "blood bag re-

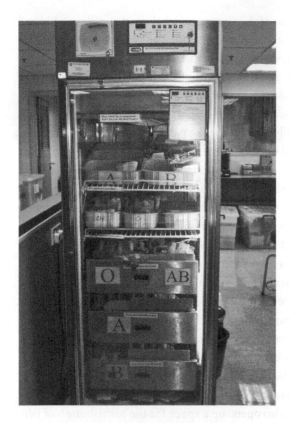

Unscreened blood is kept according to type in a refrigerator.

turned." On one occasion while I watched, an ICU nurse came down to collect blood from the blood bank. She double-checked the record book and signed it, telling me that blood was checked three times—in the book, on the patient's request form, and on the labels. It would then be checked again when it arrived on the ward. But this time the wrong bag had been brought out of the fridge where it had been put with others waiting for collection by ward staff. The MLT went to get the right one—whole blood—and changed the number and other information in the record book. She then removed plasma from the bag of whole blood as only packed cells were required for the patient. The ICU nurse told us that the patient was bleeding and they didn't know from where. She exchanged various pleasantries with the blood bank staff before taking the blood components and forms back to the ICU.

I have described some of the systems of labeling of samples and blood products that are used in the labs and blood banks. Even without an exhaustive account of these, we have seen the quite elaborate procedures in place to ensure that, however disembodied or identical to each other samples or blood components appear, they remain connected to their particular source. This is necessarily the case so that test results or screening procedures can eventually be reattached to patients or donors, or so that the source of donated blood can be verified at any point from when it has been extracted to after it has been used in transfusion. Disembodied samples moving through the lab in containers or bags of blood components, with their labels affixed to them, are thus a particular class of object—detached from persons but also indirectly attached. Because the focus of lab work is on human bodily substances, and particularly blood, and because of the multivalent qualities these samples carry, it is especially difficult to re-create them as detached and purified objects. Labels mediate between the sample or blood product and the person from whom these are derived. Like the forms that donors complete, which were considered in chapter 1, they could be seen as part of the boundary infrastructure of the labs. In outward form, samples or blood packs may be almost indistinguishable from each other, but they are also closely identifiable (unless a mix-up in the labeling procedures or the recording of information disrupts these connections), and this also opens up a space for the reattribution of personal or moral qualities.

Getting Results, Pursuing Information

I have already mentioned that when results were delayed (or even sometimes when they were not), it was quite usual for doctors or nurses to phone the lab to try to get test results quickly over the phone. It was a simple matter, then, for MLTs to go into the computer system using either the name of a patient or their hospital number to look up the results. This was part of the routine work that went on in the labs, but MLTs made clear that, by constantly reminding them of the urgency with which results were awaited, such calls contributed considerably to the stress of their work. One could also see this, however, as part of the process through which lab staff forged their own spirit of collegiality and a sense of the lab as an independent entity that ran counter to the pressure to increase workload and improve performance exerted by senior medical staff and hospital management.

That calls requesting results could potentially be problematic in other ways was brought home to me one day when I witnessed a trainee pick up a ringing phone in the blood bank when no member of the permanent staff was available. When the MLT in charge of the blood bank returned to her post, she immediately scolded the trainee. Telling him that he should not under any circumstances answer the phone, she explained that the person phoning would not necessarily realize that they were speaking to a trainee (phones in the lab were usually answered by giving the name of the department rather than the person speaking). If the caller was a doctor or someone phoning in an emergency, and instructions were rapidly conveyed without waiting for a response, the fact that a trainee was answering could lead to a misunderstanding with potentially serious consequences.

At the beginning of this chapter I described how MLTs often knew quite a lot of information about patients from whom they had taken blood on the wards. And sometimes they checked on a particular patient's progress or history out of concern or curiosity. Thus, when I was invited to observe open-heart surgery in one hospital, as described in the introduction to this book, the MLTs in the lab were able to tell me something about the patient beforehand, and how he progressed after surgery, by checking the hospital information system connected to the lab computers. But it was not just in answer to queries from me that such information might be pursued. On one occasion, while I was observing routine tests in the urinalysis department, the MLT working there expressed surprise as she was recording the results of a urine pregnancy test and noticed that the patient was sixty-six years old. Referring to the patient in recognizably Malaysian terms as "Auntie, aged 66," she said that no other tests had been requested, and added that this didn't happen very often. This initiated some joking with the two trainees who were working with her. When they asked her what the result of the test was and she told them, one of them suggested that perhaps the patient should try again. After scolding him for this levity, the MLT told the trainees that having many children can cause late menopause, while having fewer children can result in early menopause.

I was impressed by the way in which, although none of those involved had actually met the patient, a quite detailed discussion with imagined scenarios had been extrapolated from a urine sample bottle and a request form. And this recalls Singleton's (1998, 96) description of the way cervical samples are analyzed differently depending on the accompanying information on age, marital status, and number of children, and Annemarie Mol's (1998, 147–48) account of the way links between a form and a pathologist's sample may or may not be enlarged in the performance of atherosclerosis. Such links, and the hard work it takes to make them, Mol argues, contribute to the "multiple ontology" of atheroscleroses. On the day following this conversation in the lab, I asked the MLT whether she had discovered anything further about the patient. She told me she had asked around but that it had been quite difficult to find someone who knew anything. Eventually, she had discovered that the patient was part of a new research treatment using heavy radiation. For this reason, she said, they had to do a routine pregnancy test and Pap smear. She had found this out from a nurse on a third-class ward, she added. What was striking to me was the way that the MLT had of her own accord followed her curiosity and had obviously gone to some trouble out of interest derived from what she perceived as an anomaly on the request form. We might see this effort to settle an inconsistency by attributing a personal narrative to the sample as echoing the finding of Jeanette Edwards that, for her interlocutors in Bacup (in northwest England), "gametes need names" (Edwards 2000, 229–48). The name in this example signifies the importance of attributing a moral bond to embryos—as opposed to perceiving them as existing in a rootless and unhitched detachment. Thus, far from expressing the anonymity emphasized by Titmuss, the MLT's pursuit of further information about a sample and attempts to build a personal narrative seem here to invert the logic of detachment and anonymity.[4]

There were many other instances in which I heard lab staff speculate about particular patients or watched as they pursued test results on the lab computers. Tracking information in this way might sometimes be initiated by something unusual that had struck them on the request form or a test result—as in the example above—but it could also be concern about a patient whom they had encountered on the wards or among the outpatients. We can see how these apparently small and insignificant interventions rehumanize what might otherwise remain as technical tasks, detached from the lives of patients. This process of "rehumanization" affects both the content of the work done by MLTs and the results they achieve, and it is a counterpart to the process of domesticating the lab space that I described in chapter 2.[5]

Rehumanizing the work of the lab involves, as we have seen, enlarging the links between a form and a sample. One MLT spoke to me about the way that blood samples "in tubes can tell story of patient's condition. Can then check back to request form to see, and remember. Sometimes still remember [their] face, feel sorry for patient." Here we catch a glimpse of the way that, within the seemingly bounded confines of the lab, forms, samples, and results are, for staff who carry out these routine and highly technologized tests, nevertheless intrinsically connected to a patient's story. And enfolded into these connections are emotional and moral commitments.

Sometimes a desire to get to the bottom of an apparent puzzle was instrumental in achieving a diagnostic result. When I asked MLTs what gave them most satisfaction in their work, several mentioned cases of illness that had been particularly difficult to diagnose. When answering this question in an interview, one MLT recounted a case from a few years before:

> When I did my afternoon shift one time, had child's test. Child was transferred from [name of city]. [They] don't know cause of high fever. [I] noticed a malarial parasite in blood. Checked red cells—hema slide—informed ward nurse. Doctor phoned back. Was very pleased to know cause. Called me, asked for confirmation, quickly. Asked for other test—can get hemolysis with drug for malarial parasite. Some doctors very [big] ego—don't listen to MLTs. Next day, came to lab. Normally consultants don't come to lab. [She explained that she was worried as to why he had come; she thought she might be in trouble.] Brought commendation letters—one for me, one for lab manager.

Here the fact that the MLT knew the patient was a child who was seriously ill can be clearly seen to have enhanced her motivation to carry out her work as well as possible and to achieve a rapid and accurate result. In this way, the rehumanizing work carried out by the MLT—reconnecting the sample to the patient—not only increased her own interest and satisfaction, but it is also enfolded into her ethical engagement and conscientiousness. In other words, it informed and enhanced the quality of her work.

Sometimes, there were more direct connections between the results being pursued and lab staff. Partly because family members of hospital employees were eligible for treatment at reduced costs, it was not infrequent for lab staff to run tests on the samples of their relatives. In such cases, and particularly for elderly parents or grandparents, they would often try to expedite matters as simply and speedily as possible. This could mean an MLT taking the sample at home before coming to work in order to save an elderly parent having to come to the outpatient department, or getting them registered early so that they would not have to spend too long waiting. Because many of the lab staff had worked together for a long time, they were often familiar with each other's family members and would chat with them when they met in the hospital or if they came to the labs. It was therefore not just a single member of the lab staff who might be aware of their own relative's blood or other sample being tested; this knowledge would usually be shared among a number of people. It was because I was frequently told about somebody's mother or grandmother being unwell or coming for tests that I learned about these connections between colleagues. Members of staff would also help each other by looking up the results quickly. I became particularly aware of this when my daughter was sent for blood tests at one hospital and, in order to reassure me that nothing was seriously amiss, the lab staff kindly looked up her results as they appeared.

Blood and other tests and the screening of donated blood might also be necessary for members of the lab staff themselves if they donated blood, when they were unwell, as a routine health test, or after an accident in the labs. This of course meant that colleagues could easily be in possession of confidential information about each other as well as about each other's family members. I was told several times by MLTs of occasions when they had had an accident in the lab in the past that had required testing for infectious diseases. And there were of course cases of illness that were unrelated to work in the labs, which arose while I was there. No one, however, spontaneously raised worries about confidentiality among their colleagues with me, and the only time I heard the question of the confidentiality of results raised (but not in connection to test results for staff) was during a visit by a group of non-Malaysian health officials. My sense was that staff accepted this level of shared information among their colleagues as an unavoidable feature of working life and a by-product of the relations they had with each other. But one can also see this kind of shared knowledge more positively as contributing to trust and collegiality between staff members of the labs. Some of the implications of this knowledge are pursued further in the following chapter.

Although I was intrigued by the question of whether transfusion patients or members of their families ever voiced preferences for receiving blood from particular sources, the fact that my research did not focus on patients meant that I did not pursue this question directly. I touch on these matters here only insofar as they affected lab staff. Blood bank staff occasionally told me about patients who had explicitly requested that they only receive the blood of family members—indicating the ways that accepting blood might for patients be connected to kinship. I was also told by one MLT about a patient who had actually spotted from the label on a blood bag ready to be used for his transfusion that this was not the blood of the family member that had been donated specifically for his use. Staff, however, were aware that blood from family members was not necessarily likely to be more safe than that of others. As one MLT told me, "the only really safe blood is your own." And some explained that the use of autologous blood transfusion was becoming more common in scheduled surgery because it was the safest form of transfusion.

There were other accounts too which touched on the idea that specific qualities might be transferred with transfused blood. Here again we can see how the polyvalent associations of blood are difficult to expunge from the lab spaces. One MLT, for example, told me that patients sometimes commented on their skin getting darker after transfusion. She mentioned the case of a Chinese woman transfused after giving birth, who said the blood must have come from a Malay or Indian because her skin had gotten darker after the transfusion. These ideas bring into play a highly sensitive discourse relating to interethnic transfers of blood (or organs), and specifically the question of whether Muslim patients are happy to receive blood from non-Muslim donors (see Peletz 2002). We have seen how the interethnic transfer of organs was highlighted in newspaper accounts that reported the special praise of politicians for the families of donors whose gifts were seen as embodying the "harmonious spirit of Malaysia." One member of the lab staff told me that some people requested family blood because they knew about the window during which HIV infection couldn't be detected by routine screening procedures. "Some people prefer autologous transfusion," she said. But she noted that Malays donated mainly to the GH and less to private hospitals. They request Malay blood, she said, because of the prohibition on eating pork. The same MLT told me about a patient who had a low hemoglobin level; a family member had insisted on the patient getting Malay blood, and the patient had a rare blood group. "Very difficult," she commented, and added that "Chinese people mostly want family blood— fathers want sons' blood." As we spoke, I spotted a note above the reception desk in the blood bank concerning a patient for transfusion, which stated "to use own family blood." But these matters were, she said, "very sensitive in Malaysia."

It is notable that preferences for blood from Malay donors were only ever alluded to in rather hushed tones and in a manner that made clear its sensitivity by staff of the blood banks and labs during my research. Practicing Muslims apparently sometimes felt strongly that they should only receive blood from other Muslims, and might raise this issue although the Islamic authorities in Malaysia had given clear rulings that there were no concerns about Muslims receiving blood or organ donations from non-Muslims.

Conclusion

This chapter has focused on the work of the labs and some of the many intricate tasks that it entails. Although most of these tasks are quite standardized, to a considerable degree mechanized, and often routine, we have seen how there is also a space for individual variation—for example, in the way blood is taken from patients. Skill, experience, and luck are also part of work in the labs and are built into the way trainees learn to carry out procedures. Copying out standard operating procedures seems to transmit only part of what must be learned in order to carry out the work of MLTs or lab technicians—the rest must be learned by doing and by engaging with the connections between samples and patients.

In spite of high degrees of mechanization and the apparently routine aspects of work, social engagements are enfolded into even the most routinized and mechanical lab processes. We saw how the sophisticated medical technology used in the labs is humorously anthropomorphized, incorporated—at least in jest—into the kinship universe of lab sociality. And test tubes of samples or bags of blood components, which seem outwardly almost indistinguishable from each other, necessarily retain their connections to their sources of origin in specific patients or donors. While in some respects, test tubes containing samples and bags of blood components can be treated as "purified" objects that are detached from networks of relations, we have also seen that they can readily be reattached to their sources or even ascribed new moral qualities through the social interventions of lab staff or of patients. Here labels and forms have a special role as "technologies of detachment"—or reattachment—that mediate these connections but also enable them to be enlarged. When a urine sample can trigger a possible story about an unknown sixty-six-year-old "Auntie," or when Vacutainers contain the blood of a relative, friend, or colleague, we see how layered entanglements permeate the space of the labs and are in fact generated through the samples themselves. These are indeed "multiple" and unstable objects in the sense outlined by Annemarie Mol (1998, 2002), and delineating their multiplicity also illuminates the way ethics and politics are enfolded into the processes of lab work.

The propensity to rehumanize forms and samples contributes on the one hand to the instability and ambivalence of objects and knowledge in the lab to which I referred at the beginning of this chapter, but at the same time it also ensures the engagement of medical lab technologists with their work and thus improves its quality. I have suggested that the ways in which this occurs bear a similarity to the UK labs studied by Vicky Singleton, but I have also drawn attention to recognizably Malaysian idioms of sociality in the humorous use of kin terms or other modes of address that incorporate ethnic markers. The process of rehumanization requires hard work—just as its contrary process of detachment, as a form of boundary work, is also learned through work and experience. I have argued that this detachment is particularly difficult to achieve, and therefore unstable, because bodily samples, particularly blood, which originate in the bodies of patients and donors, are the material of lab work. Some of these donors and patients are known to lab staff, but even where this is not the case, moral and other qualities may be newly attributed on the basis of information available from forms or other sources.

As the opening vignette for this chapter indicated, staff are aware that trainees must learn to detach themselves from the social relations that blood encompasses. But we have seen that lab work also rests on qualities of human engagement. Both are equally intrinsic to what occurs within the spaces of the clinical pathology labs and blood banks, and both contribute to the successful outcomes of the work undertaken. Rehumanization is closely linked to the domestication of lab space, which I described in chapter 2 and pursue further in chapter 4. We could see rehumanization as material and emotional gendered labor, which contributes to the ambiguity of the lab spaces and produces particular kinds of objects and personhood. Training on the job, I suggest, not only teaches trainees the importance of detachment; it also, and contrarily, inculcates the social engagements and ethical judgments that are enfolded into lab work. Indeed, it is these aspects of their learning in the lab that trainees particularly value and enjoy. My depiction of rehumanization goes beyond the insights of Mol and of Singleton, which address the limitations of Latourian actor-network theory. Rehumanization as described here illuminates how it is through incorporating the logic of care, eating together, kinship, and home into daily working practice that the work of the labs is made stronger and more resilient. Like the morality encapsulated in naming embryos (Edwards 2000), this is a moral engagement that fractures a simple image of samples and forms as boundary objects. It indicates the multidimensional and nuanced nature of the spaces, objects, and engagements of the labs. Far from being sealed-off laboratory spaces indicated by their doorways and entry points, processes of domestication, kinship, and morality are at the heart of what goes on in these labs.

It is through rehumanizing samples and forms, sharing risks and knowledge, and domesticating the highly technologized spaces of the lab that the lab reproduces itself as a social and institutional entity. This pervasive lab sociality and ethical engagement counters the often dehumanizing tendencies of hospital management to increase workloads and improve the performance of the lab, as monitored through charts and tables displayed on the lab walls. It also runs counter to a larger logic of domaining that underlies conventional understandings of modernity (McKinnon and Cannell 2013).

The next chapter considers sociality among staff more closely. We will see how the contradictory impulses of boundary work and domestication, through which bodily samples and blood work in the labs are processed, also reflect the unresolvable tensions of these spaces. Unpicking these tensions enables us to return to some of the larger issues raised in the introduction to this book.

Medical, Supernatural,

& Moral Matters

Sightings of a *pontianak* (woman vampire) captured on video have caused a stir among locals in Malacca. · For the past fortnight, droves of people have gathered at a bridge near Jalan Pulau Gadon, Malacca, where the 50-second video-clip was purportedly filmed. · Many stayed up to the wee hours of the morning hoping to catch a glimpse of the spectre.

—"Pontianak in Malacca," *The Star*, April 15, 2008

Vampire spirits are quite commonly reported in Malaysia, and I had encountered many such stories when carrying out fieldwork in Langkawi (where they are known as *Langsuir*) in the 1980s (Carsten 1997, 124–26). Newspaper reports like the one above sometimes featured familiar local tropes of malevolent spirits and ghosts. That such spirits are undeterred by modern technology was indicated by the video clip mentioned—although it was also reported in the same article that, "as soon as the police arrived, she would turn into her true self and disappear." Stories about spirits attracted by the presence of human blood were also a feature of hospital life, and we encounter them in chapter 4.

In drawing on newspaper accounts to analyze new modes of imagined criminality that emerged in Suharto's New Order Indonesia, James Siegel (1998) argues that, in Indonesia, a domesticated set of understandings about ghosts was replaced by images and discourses of a new criminal type, which became the target for state violence and repression. Newspapers accounts, he suggests, reflect and enable new understandings of fear, criminality, rumor, ghosts, and death. Some of the qualities of ghosts that he refers to have a resonance beyond Indonesia in the regional context of Southeast Asia.[1] Stories about vampire spirits in Malaysia are often told with a kind of relish that is also palpable in newspaper accounts. Here the spectral register is part of the everyday and may be experienced in the most modern and technologically advanced contexts—including hospitals, factories, and universities. In these stories, which connect criminality, ghosts, and blood's nefarious potential, spirits are attracted by blood's animating powers. Such spirits may have murderous intentions and may also originate as the victims of murderers. These submerged resonances can be read in newspaper accounts, where blood calibrates morality and political harmony between "races" but also indicates untoward menace or criminality, or even the power of the state to counter opposition.

That security cameras and other modern forms of surveillance might fail to protect against dangers that combine human and supernatural elements was apparent in another newspaper item. "All Abuzz over Oily Man" described how students at the local university were reportedly being preyed on by an "*orang minyak* (oil man)." While "USM acting vice-chancellor Prof Ahmad Syukri Mustapa Kamal said so far the authorities had yet to receive any reports of rape or sightings by students," a "second-year communications student" told the newspaper, "Students are saying that the *orang minyak* is raping girls to improve his prowess in black magic, but whatever the reason, we are very concerned."

The same report noted, "Security has been stepped up at the entrances with closed-circuit TV camera surveillance and 24-hour patrols conducted by guards and hostel authorities."[2] Such measures, however, were not guaranteed to be effective, and we can detect an underlying register of anxiety in these accounts. I was told by staff in the hospitals where I worked that security cameras would fail to record ghosts that they had seen when they were on duty at night.

As Aihwa Ong ([1987] 2010) documented in her pioneering study of spirit possession among female Malaysian electronics factory workers in the 1980s, such stories, combining human and supernatural elements in the setting of modern, technologized institutions, are a feature of everyday urban life in Malaysia. They are reported in newspapers but are also the common currency of conversation in homes, coffee shops, and workplaces, and they encompass an explicit or implicit moral or ethical commentary on the protagonists.

In a different register, newspaper accounts less concerned with the supernatural often appeared to link, implicitly or explicitly, matters of the body to place of origin, nationality, and morality. These included local incidents—a George Town father who reportedly wanted to sell his kidney to raise money "to start a small business to feed my family," which gave his mobile phone number;[3] or a rise in the number of cases of hepatitis C in Penang.[4] Reports of foreign events were also telling: an item from the Philippines recorded that kidney transplants to foreigners had been suspended "amid allegations that poor Filipinos are being duped into selling vital organs for a pittance."[5] In Singapore, it was reported that a blood donor, "a Myanmar national," was sentenced to eight months' imprisonment "for lying about his sexual activities before donating blood subsequently found to be HIV-positive."[6] An item from Sydney reported on an Australian nine-year-old girl who, after undergoing a liver transplant, had spontaneously changed blood groups nine months later, adopting that of her donor.[7] Some reports seemed more exotic or macabre. "Group Stole 1,000 Body Parts" was the headline of another report on the trial of a male nurse in Philadelphia, who "admitted he cut body parts from 244 corpses and helped forge paperwork so the parts, some of them diseased, could be used in unsuspecting patients."[8]

The moral dimension that implicitly runs through such accounts was often apparent in more factual medical reporting too. Thus an item titled "Designer Babies Unacceptable" reported that Women, Family and Community Development Minister Datuk Dr. Ng Yen Yen had stated, "Artificial insemination of designer babies is unacceptable and is not practised in the country": "We do not wish to see a situation where people decide and design their babies. It is not ethical, she stressed, adding that such a situation could only occur if it was proven that there were serious genetic difficulties resulting in death for the unborn child."[9] In spite of the minister's assertion, quoted in the same article, that "we are very particular about sex selection as well," advertisements for sex-selection procedures appeared in newspapers, and these services were privately obtainable.

In a short article recording the first official celebration of International AIDS Memorial Day, the Deputy Health Minister was reported to have advised, "Every woman should carry a condom for her own protection." The article gave Health Ministry figures for the numbers of women (but not men) who contracted HIV infection between 2000 and 2007 and continued, "Malaysian AIDS Council (MAC) president, Prof Dr Adeeba Kamarulzaman said apart from sex workers, a large number of women who contracted HIV were housewives, infected unknowingly by their husbands who could be drug addicts."[10] Dr. Adeeba was reported to have said that, in spite of knowing about the protective value of condoms, "there are some men who do not care to take precautions, even though they know they have HIV, and they don't tell their wives." Having thus indicated gendered distinctions between the moral worth of different categories of men and women infected with HIV, the article concluded by giving the Health Ministry figures of the number of "HIV sufferers" for "Malays," "Chinese," "Indians," and "foreigners."

Another genre of newspaper reports, which appeared regularly, as they do in many other parts of the world, consisted of feature articles on matters of health, often as a regular health supplement, and including advice from doctors about regular testing or diet. An article on "The Kidney and Blood Pressure Link" (*The Star*, May 8, 2008) was published "in conjunction with World Hypertension Day" and was provided "courtesy of NKF KIDNEY CARE, a community education programme by National Kidney Foundation of Malaysia." Printed in *The Star*'s weekly "Fit4life" supplement, it discussed how high blood pressure could damage the kidneys and the importance of having blood pressure as well as kidney function measured regularly. A feature article, by Dr. Milton Lum, "chairperson of the Commonwealth Medical Trust," published in the same supplement, warned about the potential negative effects of a rise in preventive health checks and screening tests, and the phenomenon of the "worried well."[11] Such items indicate the expanding middle-class and urban demographics of Malaysia that we encountered in chapter 2 and correlate the implications for health care.

Sometimes such articles focused on particular conditions, or new treatments, or on wider issues of social concern. Medical reporting often included policy issues concerning medical payments. A two-page spread on "Hospital Charges and Fee Splitting," also by Dr. Milton Lum, informed readers about the basis for private hospitals' charges. These were composed of two elements: doctors' fees and hospital charges.

The doctors' professional fees include consultation fees, fees for ward visits and procedure fees.

The hospital charges include accommodation, laboratory, imaging, medication, labour ward, operating theatre, nursing, physiotherapy and other charges.

The article went on to explain the importance of this distinction:

Doctors' professional fees are regulated by the Private Healthcare Facilities and Services Act (PHFSA) and its regulations.

However, the charges of private hospitals are unregulated, for reasons best known to the powers-that-be involved in the formulation of the Regulations of the PHFSA.[12]

Articles such as these might have a strong ethical theme—in this case focused on the practice of "fee-splitting" (charging for referrals between medical practitioners, which contravenes the PHFSA) and on the growing importance of "healthcare middlemen" (commercial companies). The same article also discussed whether hospital discounts, which might be offered to insurance companies, managed care corporations, and corporate organizations in return for a large volume of purchased services, were actually in the interests of patients. We saw in chapter 1 how this kind of public concern is also reflected in donors' worries about the possibility that blood, which had been freely given, might be charged for in private hospitals—an anxiety that raises issues of trust and that doctors are anxious to dispel.

Alongside such feature articles, the intensity of commercial interests surrounding medical care was also demonstrated by advertisements for various kinds of health care products. Cervical cancer vaccination, vitamin and other dietary supplements, and herbal remedies for colds were among the items frequently promoted. Some of the products seemed outlandish: an advertisement for Thomson Livrin 300 suggested that the "300 mg of standardised Milk Thistle Extract with 80% silymarin from Switzerland" would "help support liver functions" and, by implication, help "to remove harmful and toxic substances from our blood." Thomson's OsteoPro, containing "fully reacted Glucosamine Sulfate (non-shellfish) from USA," "Lubricates and Restores Joint Mobility."

Sometimes it was the juxtaposition of products as much as the items themselves that attracted attention. In one newspaper, an advertisement declaring "BABY BOY or BABY GIRL. Now you can choose" showed a picture of a handsome baby and promised "100% Money back Guarantee." The procedure was claimed as a "breakthrough technology from France," that was "scientifically proven with a success rate of 98.7% by Prokiad International Laboratory." Immediately adjacent on one side was an advertisement for a seminar on psoriasis and eczema and, on the other, for "Hongshang HEAT SHRINKABLE PRODUCTS"—whose exact purpose was unclear, but apparently it was something electrical. As in many parts of the world, in Malaysia such unexpected contiguities are often the source of jokes and humor. Perhaps surprisingly, as we see in the following chapter, the labs and those who worked in them were also the sites and users of such different kinds of medical treatment.

The language of these promotions suggests the enhanced power and effectiveness of foreign medical technologies and products. When one private hospital in Penang gained international accreditation for 2008–10 from the Joint Commission International (JCI), the opportunity was taken to run three full pages of advertisements in *The Star*, together with several medical technology companies, recording this achievement.[13] Three snapshots of hospital life featured in each advertisement showed various high-tech aspects of medical care (computers, ultrasound images, a procedure in an operating room) and a smiling and uniformed multiethnic medical care team. The prominence of non–locally sourced materials, or the "international," in these advertisements as sources of high-quality health care is reminiscent of the "foreign medical experts" who featured in the newspaper reports on the treatment of Anwar Ibrahim's blood sample cited earlier.

Media accounts of Anwar Ibrahim's case had dramatically highlighted how the issue of trust—in the state, in the police, in legal and hospital procedures—cannot be divorced from the substance of social relations. While the state in that case asserted the effectiveness of independent scientific processes as guarantor of the integrity of these procedures, Anwar sought to undermine the state's authority by upholding the centrality of social relations to how the results were obtained and what they might imply. If his sample had been tampered with, social relations were at issue. We saw how blood donors too voiced issues of trust in their decisions over which hospitals to donate to, and doctors in Penang were acutely sensitive to newspaper accounts that imputed the trust of the public to the social relations of blood donation.

Returning to the supernatural register with which this section began, it seems hardly coincidental that newspapers articulate a set of associations made between blood, death, dirt, danger, and ghosts to which everyday life in modern institutions may be exposed. They suggest underlying anxieties that focus on trust and the possibility of corruption. In chapter 4 we find such associations articulated by staff within the clinical pathology labs and explore the anxieties and dangers they calibrate.

FOUR

"Work Is Just *Part* of the Job"

Ghosts, Food, and Relatedness in the Labs

I had been observing life in the clinical pathology labs and blood banks for three or four months before I began to notice the ghosts. Having become apparent, however, they seemed hard to avoid. One morning in the blood bank, I was talking to Sharon, one of the medical lab technologists, as she was preparing equipment to take on a mobile blood campaign the following Sunday. Sharon mentioned that she herself wouldn't be able to attend the blood drive, as she would be on call in the lab. She preferred blood campaigns to being on call, she said, because the latter meant being on duty at night. When I asked whether she slept at the lab, Sharon said she didn't—she was scared to because of the ghosts. Were there ghosts in the blood bank? I asked. On this matter Sharon's reply was equivocal: "Temporarily, it's OK," she said.

The first account I heard of ghosts concerned an unsettling set of events at the house of the recently deceased grandmother of one of the lab trainees where relatives had gathered the night before the funeral. Such stories, told with considerable relish and excitement, would often trigger longer discussions, to which others would contribute their experiences of uncanny events—some of which had nothing to do with the hospital, labs, or blood banks. As I listened more closely, however, I caught traces of ghostly presences within the workspaces of the labs and blood banks. One day, I heard one of the senior MLTs, Li Ann, telling a small group of trainees about working in the hospital: the different kinds of work available and the opportunities for training; the importance of time management, shifts, and on-call duty; and how they should not listen to ghost stories. I interjected a query about ghosts in the lab, and Li Ann said there were no ghosts in the present lab but, yes, in the old one she had "felt the presence of evil."

Others were more matter-of-fact. One medical lab technologist reported that she would "normally [turn] on the radio and listen to music" when she felt something strange going on at night. Several agreed that ghosts had been prone to appear in the lab's old premises in the hospital but, when they had moved upstairs some months before, things had improved. In the old lab downstairs, another medical lab technologist, Kamariah, told me she had once heard a little girl laughing. When she went to look, a little girl was jumping over a drain, playing. Kamariah said she had looked at the clock; it was 3:00 a.m. She shut the door and turned up the radio. Normally, she said, she didn't listen to the radio. Downstairs was dirty, Kamariah added, and also it was open to the outside and to thieves.

One afternoon, as I was talking to someone in the immunology department, I noticed an animated discussion on the other side of the lab where several MLTs and a medical perfusionist were gathered around a workbench. When I went to investigate, I found them excitedly discussing how an Indian nurse had apparently seen a headless man in the old building of the hospital. The perfusionist brought up another story of a patient who had requested a transfer from a third-class ward to a first-class one because noise had prevented him from sleeping. He was given a separate room but, because during the night he had felt children playing with his feet, he had abandoned the room to sit at the nurses' station instead. Another patient, the perfusionist related, an Indian lawyer, had also complained about children running around in the night. I asked whether there were ghosts here in the lab, and he replied that there weren't any yet, but they were close by. And also, he added, "The blood bank is here." I asked whether ghosts were attracted by the blood bank. They were, he replied, and went on to tell me about the ghosts of women patients who had "hung themselves using their own blouses in psychy ward toilets."

● ● ●

The hospital blood banks and clinical pathology labs were, as we saw in chapter 2, highly technologized working environments. The main part of these workspaces was closed to patients and members of the public, and this was made clear by notices at the entrances to these departments. The working environments were air-conditioned, calm, and quiet, as white-coated medical lab technologists engaged in a multitude of different detailed tasks associated with blood grouping, diagnostic testing, screening, and cross-matching. So what kinds of entities were these ghosts? And what attributes of social relations might their presence indicate?

This chapter focuses on some of the seemingly small ways in which "laboratory life" and everyday life in Penang coexist in the lab. In the main parts of the chapter I describe how those who work in the clinical pathology labs and blood banks endeavor to make these spaces sociable. Within this highly technologized working environment we can discern a process of "domestication"—involving food, friendships, and kin relations—that is set in motion by the medical laboratory technologists and lab technicians who work there. But apart from delineating the *forms* of this sociality, I also want to suggest how they matter. The stories presented here are ones in which the boundaries between the lab, the blood bank, and the world outside seem unclear or fuzzy. There are, of course, several levels on which this might be significant. One is how such "boundary crossings" affect the working lives of lab technicians and medical lab technologists; another is what they indicate more generally about how these employees experience the work processes that go on in these spaces; and a third might be what they tell us even more generally about social relations in Malaysia.

We saw in chapter 3 how, as they go about their work, medical lab technologists and lab technicians have a tendency to "rehumanize" the forms and samples that they encounter. In this chapter I argue that this rehumanization occurs alongside other processes of domestication, and this suggests the possibility of at least of some "uneven seepage," to use Rayna Rapp's term, "in the traffic between biomedical and familial discourses" (Rapp 1999, 303; see also Lock et al. 2006). Just what is meant by seepage? For the moment, I suggest that the circulation of different kinds and idioms of sociality in these spaces reveals how the separations between "laboratory life" and "everyday life" in Penang are uneven and incomplete. Such idioms and forms of identification circulate in the same spaces, sometimes directly colliding, often apparently coexisting, without necessarily having obvious consequences for work practices. This, in turn, might lead us to reflect not only on the nature of "domaining practices" central to kinship as an analytic field—and to its assumed isolation within a domestic sphere in modern societies—but also on the related symbolic importance of science as a "sacred domain" that "supposedly transcend[s] human agency" (Yanagisako and Delaney 1995, 13; see also Carsten 2004; Schneider 1984).

In terms of scientific practice, Latour and others have argued that "laboratory life" proceeds *as if* it were wholly separate from the rest of life, and that "the work of purification," which is central to the lab, involves separating nature and society, but that this is a pretense because in reality, nature is actually *constructed* rather than *discovered* in the laboratory (Latour 1993, 30–31). The connections between nature and society—the denial of which Latour suggests is crucial to the project of modernity—are actually central to how science works. The presumed isolation of kinship within a domestic sphere and its separation from such pursuits as scientific and laboratory work are seen as equally foundational to the project of modernity (see McKinnon and Cannell 2013). The co-occurrence of a world of kinship and other modes of sociality alongside a rigorously enforced regime of laboratory work suggests, at the very least, some fractures and wobbles, some gentle mergings and crisscrossings, between these supposedly separate domains. As we saw in the previous chapter, following Singleton (1998), the rehumanization of samples in the labs is not merely incidental to what goes on in the labs but actually intrinsic to maintaining the interest of those who work in them and to the high quality of their work. But domestication may not necessarily be a smooth or unproblematic process. Having delineated some of the contours of sociality among staff in the labs and blood banks, in the final parts of this chapter I return to the matter of ghosts and probe the untoward significance of their presence. I argue that this can be seen as an expression of both the perceived risks of these workspaces and of the connection between blood and animation. In my conclusion I return to the larger questions about purification, modernity, and domaining that are raised by this ethnography.

Convivial Relations

During the time I spent in Penang, I tried to establish what kinds of social connections existed among the staff working in the clinical pathology labs and between these workers and staff in other departments of the same hospitals. I built up a sense of people's lives through their work and through the kinds of things that people talk about with their colleagues. Some of these colleagues had known each other for a very long time; they were also friends, or even spouses, and they could often tell me about each other.

There were many incidents in the everyday running of the labs that revealed quite a lot about the family lives, backgrounds, concerns, and opinions of staff on matters that went beyond the workplace. I had the sense that what I was learning was quite fragmentary—in the same way that, in many contemporary institutions, what we know about most of our colleagues is often fragmentary. By placing some of these vignettes side by side, it is nevertheless possible to build up a sense of the texture of the lives and social relations of those I studied.

Much of what I learned was in one way or another over food. Food, as any Penangite will relate, is an important part of life on the island. Penang is renowned for its wonderfully diverse culinary culture (encompassing Chinese, Malay, Indian, and Western cooking traditions among others) and the huge number of excellent restaurants and hawker stalls. People in Penang love to talk about food, and do so constantly, swapping recipes and recommendations about favorite eateries. Food is, of course, not allowed in the lab, and this prohibition was displayed on the walls of labs, where, as we saw in chapter 2, eating areas were strictly separated from work areas. It thus seemed paradoxical to discover the degree to which food was a fundamental part of collegial relations and a major topic of conversation. The clinical pathology labs that I studied had areas separated from the workspaces where staff could bring food and eat. In one lab this was a small table and seating area screened off at the end of the main laboratory space and equipped with a fridge, sink, and kettle. In another, it was part of an outside area adjacent to the labs and connected to a storeroom and an on-call room where staff could sleep or rest. This space, also equipped for very simple cooking, had been made pleasant, as described in chapter 2, by an elaborate arrangement of plants and a series of fishponds with running water between them that had been constructed and maintained by some of the lab staff.

The eating areas in both labs were well used by the staff. Some would bring breakfast and eat there before starting work in the mornings; some would bring food from home or outside stalls or from the hospital canteen and eat there at lunchtime. Drinks could be made on the spot using kettles or could be brought in. Quite often someone would bring in a special snack—such as fruit, biscuits, or cake—that could be shared with colleagues; this was especially true during the major festivals like Chinese New Year. Lab staff would also go in groups to eat lunch together—either to the hospital canteen, to outside stalls not far from the hospital, or occasionally to a reasonably priced restaurant. These groups of two or three colleagues, or sometimes more, took their customary form, and I would join with some of them. Because the same colleagues tended to eat together regularly, I too was quite quickly absorbed into these habitual commensal patterns.

On an informal and spontaneous basis, small groups of friends would sometimes go out together in the evenings—to see a film, eat a meal in a restaurant, or go to a karaoke bar. These events tended to involve younger, unmarried staff and especially those without young children. Occasionally, there were more formal eating occasions organized by the lab staff. Until relatively recently, I was told by the staff in one of the labs, they had once a year cooked a large meal outside together. In another lab, I was told that, in the past, senior staff might have organized this kind of annual event in their own homes. Large celebratory events away from the lab were considered somewhat difficult to organize because of the requirements of shift work or on-call duties, which made it impossible for all staff to attend. But there were also ways around these constraints. Biotech companies installing large, expensive items of equipment might be encouraged to order in a meal for the lab, which would take a recognizable Malaysian form, or food would be ordered in to mark a colleague leaving for a new job. The choice of menu would be a matter of much discussion and some anxiety for the organizer. For occasions when all the lab staff were involved, the menu had to take account of different dietary restrictions—especially the Muslim prohibition of pork—although the majority of the staff was Malaysian Chinese. This is an accepted part of contemporary Malaysian life in ethnically diverse settings.

Thus, although it is true to say that food was not allowed in the lab, one could also say that relations between colleagues were established and maintained through everyday and more festive commensality. This might involve something as simple as a shared bag of mangos brought from a visit to parents in the village, or a box of biscuits baked at home, or perhaps something more elaborate like a full meal involving a small group of friends or even the entire staff of the lab. When a succession of batches of young student trainees arrived over a period of weeks in one of the labs I studied, they would at first go to eat lunch together. But gradually the trainees established tentative commensal relations with the permanent staff, and groupings were established through gender, age, ethnic, or other connections, sometimes crisscrossing these in different ways.

Food and commensality thus marked spatial as well as social separations of the hospital and the labs: one could eat in the hospital canteen with other hospital staff or eat in the designated space attached to the labs that was only available to clinical pathology and blood bank staff; one could go out to eat at lunch or (more rarely) in the evening with one's chosen group of friends; and one could bring home-cooked or home-grown food or produce to work, either for sharing or to eat alone. In any case, staff would wash their hands at the designated sinks in view of colleagues after finishing their work and before eating. Occasionally it was possible to observe seepages at the boundaries between eating and noneating areas of the lab. A special meal ordered in to a "clean" meeting room that was too small for all staff might necessitate some people colonizing the manager's office or other work spaces to eat; occasionally, a few sweets or a small snack might be quickly eaten in a work area but not at a lab bench or space where samples were collected.

There were some groups of workplace friends who would eat together almost every day; others were more flexible in their eating arrangements. It was noticeable too that those who regularly ate together were often of the same ethnicity (and this could partly be explained teleologically through different ethnic food proscriptions)—though once again one could also regularly detect seepages across ethnic lines. Since co-eating was a mark of friendship and, as I myself experienced, also initiated friendships, temporality was folded into commensal work relations. Collegiality could be transformed from something transient into warm friendship through regular co-eating and, conversely, fractures in work friendships were also marked through the cessation of such relations. Sometimes, as I describe below, co-eating could be transformed into more long-lasting ties involving household members or even marriage.

Food thus marked spatial, social, and ethnic separations and seepages; it was an indicator of cleanliness and purity; it was a barometer of the warmth and strength of connections; it articulated temporal accretions and fractures among colleagues.[1] In short, as many anthropologists have described (Appadurai 1981; Carsten 1997; Douglas 1966), it was a kind of moral barometer of social relations.

Laboratory Connections

It was over lunch with small groups of colleagues that I learned many of the most interesting things about the lives of staff in the clinical pathology labs and blood banks. On one occasion, over a Kentucky Fried Chicken lunch,[2] I asked one young couple, a medical lab technologist and a hospital administrator, how they had originally gotten together. With some laughter and embarrassment, Stephen, the young man from the human resources department, first told me to ask Mr. Khoo, the lab manager. But he then related how Mr. Khoo had invited him to come on a mobile blood drive four years previously. About a month after this event, Stephen told me, he asked his fiancée-to-be out on a date. Blood donation campaigns, as we saw in chapter 1, are serious work events, but they sometimes have the air of an office outing because they involve going in a group of ten or more staff in hospital vehicles to places outside the hospital, such as temples, factories, Chinese association halls, or shopping malls. These may be elsewhere on the island or some distance away on the mainland. Such excursions may take most of the day and can involve a lunch along the way. Stephen told me that Mr. Khoo now claims he arranged their match. I asked him whether he knew he was being set up before he went on the blood drive, and he told me he did. Meanwhile, his partner was looking more and more surprised as she listened to this exchange. She told me that, until I asked about it, she hadn't heard that her fiancé knew about the matchmaking intentions of her boss before their first meeting—although she had known that her boss was somehow involved. This young couple was planning their wedding a few months hence, and it was expected that, as when others in the lab held their wedding celebrations, they would invite all their colleagues.

Over the months I was there, I came to know of several marriage relations involving staff from the lab with staff from other departments. There were also quite a few people who had other relatives, distant or closer—in one case a brother, in another a mother—working elsewhere in the same hospital. In one of the hospitals this was so much the case that I was advised never to say anything about staff working elsewhere in the same hospital just in case it turned out to concern a relative of the person to whom I was talking. One senior medical lab technologist was married to a colleague in the same lab; another's husband had previously worked in the same lab but he had recently left the hospital to take up further studies. Although it took me some time to learn about these connections, they were not particularly hard to find when I started looking. In the case of the brothers who somehow kept popping up in each other's departments, it was in fact hard to miss—especially after the one who worked in physiotherapy came to donate blood in the blood bank while his brother was working close by.

Children and babies were another source of connection between staff. They were often the subject of conversations between colleagues who would relate problems they were having to each other, issues about feeding and diet, funny stories, or achievements of their children. During lulls in working hours, they also often showed each other recent pictures of their children, which they carried on their cell phones. Babies were regularly brought into the hospital for health checks and blood tests, which were available to staff at reduced rates, and so they might be brought to greet colleagues in the lab. Similarly, elderly parents of staff were eligible for treatment at reduced rates at the hospital, so colleagues were usually familiar with each other's parents, spouses, and children.

Medical lab technologists and other staff in clinical pathology labs and blood banks often talked about their own and family members' ailments and possible cures in terms of the different kinds of medical knowledge (Chinese, Ayurvedic, and Malay) that circulate in Malaysia. Some of these conversations and references were quite fleeting and cropped up when a relative was ill or somebody had back pain or the flu. Different ways of dealing with these everyday problems might then be discussed with colleagues and, depending on background and the nature of the problem, a Chinese remedy for sore throat or a particularly skilled specialist in Chinese massage might be recommended.

A more consistent theme in discussions about health matters related to babies and childbirth. Many of the medical lab technologists were, as we saw in chapter 2, married women with young children. When I asked them individually about their experiences of childbirth, I was surprised to learn that almost all of them had gone through a lengthy period of postnatal restrictions and taboos involving special diet, restrictions on bathing, and the application of heat to their stomach. These practices are very widespread in Malaysia, and I encountered the Malay version of them in the 1980s when carrying out fieldwork in a rural Malay village (Carsten 1995b, 1997).[3] In urban contexts in contemporary Malaysia, it is common to hear middle-class people talk of a period of "confinement" (using the English term) after childbirth, and in Penang there are a number of private "confinement homes" where women can spend this period if it is more convenient than being looked after at home. The women I asked in the labs, however, spoke about being under the care of their mother-in-law or their mother during confinement, and often attributed the fact that they followed these restrictions to the strictness of their senior kin.

One reason I had not expected medical lab technologists working in clinical pathology labs to follow these postnatal practices is that, in both the Malay and the Chinese cases, they focus on matters to do with "wind" and blood—precisely their area of technical or scientific expertise. The central idea is that giving birth involves the loss of blood and is a "cooling" process. This means that after giving birth, in order to restore the body to its normal state, women should stay in the house and should avoid various kinds of food that are thought to be "cooling" (especially raw fruit and vegetables and iced drinks). In the Chinese case, I was told by lab staff, ginger is thought to be good for heating and red dates for restoring the blood. Women should also avoid bathing in cold water; they bathe in warm water to which various herbs have been added, and they may have heat applied in various ways to their body or to their stomach. The period of confinement is arduous in a tropical climate because it lasts for forty-four days in the Malay case and at least one month, I was told, in the Chinese, and it involves subjecting the body to heat. One medical lab technologist, Jo Wee, told me that she had followed these prohibitions but hadn't enjoyed it. She couldn't wash her hair for a month and had to use alcohol, so that it would evaporate, and herbs. "But," she said, "it works." To indicate their efficacy, Jo Wee referred to a colleague of hers who hadn't followed the proper restrictions and now had a problem with backache. However, she told me that she thought her daughter's generation wouldn't do it—she had already wavered. Jo Wee asked me about scientific proof for these ideas, and then told me that Chinese people also worry about "wind" (using the Malay term, *masuk angin*, literally, "wind enters"). She then asked me what I had done after giving birth. Did I wash my hair? When I said that I did, she nodded and said, "Maybe Chinese more susceptible." We agreed that these were somewhat mysterious matters.

There were many different ways then for kinship and other types of close relations to be the basis of connections between staff who worked in the blood banks and clinical pathology labs. Sometimes these connections might be quite loose—such as the shared health concerns of women who have young children. Or they could be the kind of connection that builds up gradually between colleagues who have worked together over several decades, developing mutual interests that might be invested in projects like the construction and daily maintenance of a set of decorative fishponds at the labs and involving visits to each other's houses. In one case of colleagues who had worked together over a very long period, one of them had lodged for some time many years previously in the other's parental home. Sometimes the connections were direct and intimate—leading to marriage between colleagues within the lab in two cases I knew of, and in another to an engagement between a member of staff and a young woman who had formerly been a trainee in the lab.

In the labs and blood banks that I observed it seemed to me that relations were in many ways warm and usually harmonious—although one lab appeared to have more obvious friction between colleagues. This was manifested in a general concern about "groupings" or cliques, and although this was not explicitly articulated in terms of ethnic differences, it seemed to me that this potentiality was present. This was partly because such distinctions to some degree underlay commensal patterns between colleagues. My impression was that there was a higher "density" of social relations than one might find in similar Western settings, and that this partly resulted both from the considerable length of time that many colleagues had been working together and from locally accepted cultural practices and norms.

If food was a way to initiate friendships between colleagues and underlay temporal accretions and fractures in social relations, over time it could also provide an avenue to transform collegial relations into bonds of kinship. The manner in which such transformations could occur was recognizably Malaysian (without necessarily being exclusive to Malaysia)—an insistence on sociability and a strong curiosity and interest in different kinds of food and ways of cooking that could sometimes travel across ethnic boundaries. The density of sociality, and the instances recounted to me in which workplace conviviality had been transformed over time into marital relations, reminded me of the forms of sociability that I had encountered among

Malay villagers in Langkawi in the 1980s, where eating proper rice meals together over time created bonds of kinship (Carsten 1995b, 1997). Analogies between Indian, Chinese, and Malay ideas connecting food consumption, the body, and ties between persons suggest their translatability (see Appadurai 1981; Daniel 1984; Lambert 2000; Marriott 1976; Stafford 2000; S. Thompson 1988). Despite the fact that food here, as in many ethnically plural urban settings in Malaysia, is an obvious marker of ethnic boundaries and, over time, can solidify and entrench "groupings" in the workplace, I suggest that it is also a potential means of overcoming them—both temporarily and more permanently. And this ambivalence perhaps explains why food consumption in such settings is the subject of considerable anxiety.

The symbolic potential of shared consumption in this case had a further twist in that those who worked in the blood banks and clinical pathology labs, like other hospital staff, were strongly encouraged to donate blood to the hospital blood bank in order to maintain supplies there. And quite regularly they persuaded their spouses, boyfriends or girlfriends, and connections elsewhere in the hospital to come to the blood banks to do so. Thus it was not uncommon to find one colleague taking blood from another or from the spouse of a colleague in the blood bank. One might thus speak of a process of domestication of the workspace that could have transformative potential for bodies and kin relations, and which operated not just through the sharing of meals, friendships, time, and conviviality but also, and in a unique completion of this cycle, through the shared donation of blood to the hospital blood bank. I argue that this gradual thickening of relations over time is a crucial dimension of the ethical and moral engagement of those who work in the labs, their gendered labor, and the kind of domestication at work. This domestication, parallel with the rehumanization we saw in the previous chapter, indicates that the world of the labs, rather than being rigidly bounded, is part of the world outside and of modern life in Penang more generally. Domestication, in other words, is not here a binary process occurring in opposition to work but intrinsic to it.

Laboratory Lives

The interpenetration of work with other forms of sociality was not restricted to a register of commensality or kinship; it also took more explicitly ethical or religious forms. Anne was one of the older staff members in the lab where she worked. She was in her fifties when I interviewed her and had been working as a laboratory technician, and then senior lab technician, in the hospital for more than twenty years. Her main job was as a phlebotomist—she worked in the outpatients section of the department, taking blood from outpatients who were referred there for blood tests by doctors at the hospital. Anne was unmarried and had no children. Her parents were no longer living, but she often told me about her nieces and nephews, whose lives she followed with great interest. When I asked her what had originally made her go into her field of work, Anne said, "I'm a Christian. After I left school . . . I wanted to go to England to follow my sister [who was working there]. I prayed, asked for God's direction. I felt I was going to do something medical. I wanted to do nursing."

When I asked Anne what she most enjoyed about her work, she told me a rather remarkable story. The manner in which she related it made clear that it was of central importance to her. I reproduce it here as I noted it down at the time:

> In my prayers I ask, "What is the purpose of my being here so long? Stagnating here." [Here she talked about how she had been working at the hospital for some years already and was bored and depressed.]
>
> One patient came. From Jakarta. She came once in the morning. I was busy and didn't have time to talk to her. Then she came a second time in the afternoon—[I was] more free. She had had chemo already. I asked her name. She told me. I said, "That's a very unique name." [The name combined different ethnic elements in an unusual way.] She broke down and cried. I was so shocked. I said, "What happened to you?" She told me that she had been here before—less than three months before, she had had an operation. Now the doctor said she needed a second operation straight away—not to wait at all; she needed to have it now. She was not prepared for this. Her sister and relatives had come with her; they were not prepared. Sister had to go home. All had to go home. She said, "I'm not prepared." Then suddenly I heard a voice: "visit her." I turned around and told her "I'll visit you." I asked if she needs anything. I said, "I'll visit you tonight." I was working, and said I would visit when I got off work. After work I went to the supermarket, got a box of cornflakes,

so that she would have what she needed in the morning. Then I went to see her. [I] said, "I told you I would come after work when I was free." I gave her the cornflakes. She wanted to pay me. I said, "Just accept it as a Christmas present"—it was that time in December. So she asked me, "Are you a Christian?" I was struggling to start a conversation—we're both strangers. I don't know what to do, what to say. I should share with her. [Here Anne reiterated how difficult she found this at the time.] She worshipped the Goddess of Mercy. Her sister was Christian, she wasn't. Her sister had been trying to persuade her to convert but she didn't. She prayed to Jesus, "If you are there, send someone, send an angel or whatever." She said to me, "Oh you are sent." Operation was the next day. Then chemo in Penang. She couldn't go back to Jakarta. We became friends. She stayed with me. She is still well, phones from time to time.

She shared with me instead of me sharing with her. I was supposed to share with her but she shared with me. Then I found God has a purpose.

Sometimes find nice patients; sometimes not nice ones.

When I asked Anne about connections between her work and her home life, once again religion came in. She told me that she belonged to the Medical Christian Fellowship, an organization that carries out health screenings and other charitable services. She said,

So, it is connected; also connects to family. When my mum fell sick, I realized she had a kidney problem. . . . I like talking to patients—like the Warfarin one who came this morning [referring to an older woman patient whom I had noticed she spent some time chatting to]. She's been many times to have Warfarin level checked—once had to be admitted with serious bleeding.

The central motif in this conversation was about religious experience and how it gives meaning to Anne's life—but it was significant that the epiphanic moment for her had occurred at work. So work, religion, and personal life were strongly connected, and her family life was placed in the background, which perhaps connects to her never having married. Although the majority of the medical lab technologists and lab technicians whom I interviewed did not talk to me extensively about their religious beliefs or activities, a few others did spontaneously speak about the importance of religion in their lives. Kamariah was a Malay Muslim woman in her thirties, married and with a baby, who had been working as an MLT for seven years. Thoughtful, sociable, and lively, she had originally come to work in the hospital in the 1990s as a lab technician before being sent for training as an MLT. When I asked her what had originally drawn her into her chosen career, she said, "I like to serve; very interested in that." She described to me how at school she had been active in clubs, "serving the people," as she put it. She had wanted to do a nursing course but at the time, she told me, nurses at this hospital weren't allowed to wear trousers; they had to wear a "skirt and no *tudung*" [Muslim head covering]. "I can't do that," she said. Kamariah was a member of the breast cancer support group in the hospital and did hospital visiting at the main public hospital in Penang. She was an active participant in hospital staff outings and social activities. Kamariah also told me about her husband's difficulties finding a post as an Islamic teacher in Penang and how they wanted to move to somewhere on the mainland. She said Penang was not a good Muslim environment for her son and that she and her husband wanted to bring him up in a Muslim community.

Somewhat to my surprise, directly following this, Kamariah spoke about how she had learned scuba diving on a three-month, full-time course on the east coast of Malaysia and was part of Penang's emergency search and rescue team. She explained that this meant diving to retrieve dead bodies—people who have jumped from Penang Bridge. Kamariah told me the rescue service only has two women divers. Most of these suicide attempts, she said, occur in February—"Valentine's Day—love. And exam results." She said this too was part of her service ethic—"serve whole life," she said. The ethics of Islam and service were central here, but they emerged in unpredictable ways. Kamariah, like a few other MLTs, mentioned that originally she had wanted to go into nursing, and this seemed to be directly linked to her ethical and religious orientation. It was also reflected in her daily interactions with hospital patients: when I observed her taking blood, she often spent time talking to patients.

My third example of this kind of entanglement between work and ethical aspects of life is Li Ann. In her thirties, married, and with three young children, Li Ann was a relatively senior person in the lab. Outgoing, warm, and highly intelligent, she had a degree in biochemistry and microbiology and had been working as a medical lab technologist for fifteen years. Li Ann was a Baptist Christian, and her husband was a pastor. She told me that she accompanied her husband when he went preaching and that sometimes he engaged in charismatic healing.

When I asked Li Ann how she had come to take up her particular line of work, she said, "I just want[ed] to work in hospital environment because both parents working in hospital. Growing up, stayed in hospital quarters. So it's just family-lah! Always wanted to be in hospital. Since studied science, had to be in lab." Li Ann's mother and sister were nurses, and her father had also worked in a hospital before his retirement.

Li Ann was always concerned about colleagues, and especially about the young trainees who were carrying out internships in the lab. These concerns, however, were not restricted to work matters. It was not unusual to find her in deep discussion at her lab bench with her assigned trainees. But if one listened closely to the topics of these conversations, they were as likely to feature advice about family matters, choosing a spouse, their careers, financial affairs, or medical insurance as to be instruction in the technical matters of testing for lupus, HIV, or syphilis. One day, while she was running some immunology tests on blood samples and we were talking, Li Ann told me that she often wakes up early in the morning and reads. I asked her what she liked to read. "The Bible and finance," she replied and continued, "Actually there's a lot about finance in the Bible—how to manage, planning, partners, finance." Then she began talking about marriage and about how finance is a very important factor in divorce: "People have unreal expectations," she said. "Husbands spend a lot, gamble." She said that she tells the trainees about finance and personal matters and that it's very important for them to learn. Finance, she said, was "the most important thing in marriage because it can lead to bad relations. The machines are all different in different labs, but this stuff, relations, personal stuff, is the same." On another occasion she told me, "Actually, work is all the same, it's the people that make a difference, are interesting."

Li Ann clearly saw her role in the trainees' education as one of counselor—an adviser on life and relationships—rather than just an instructor on specific aspects of the job. And this attitude was fully reciprocated by the trainees themselves. When I asked Zunirah, who had been rotating between different sections of the lab over some weeks, which department she liked best, she immediately said, "Immunology. Because Madam Tan [Li Ann] gives advice—about saving, insurance. Advises to buy house, a car. Very useful." So, a question about work and departments was transformed into one about quite other matters. Referencing other sections of the lab she had enjoyed working in, including Kamariah's, Zunirah said, "I like the people."

On another occasion I heard Li Ann quizzing a small group of trainees about tests for hepatitis B and C and premarital blood screening. The topic under discussion, however, was not the technicalities of these procedures but what the trainees themselves would do if confronted with positive results of a boyfriend or girlfriend. Later, I asked Li Ann why she was talking to trainees about this. She said it was to "find out their seriousness." She told me that the nature of marriage, and attitudes toward it, has changed. "Now young people don't take it seriously. They sleep around, don't look after their health. Marriage is not just about sex," she said; it is "about commitment," and today, the young "just marry—without proper commitment." Li Ann told me she wanted the trainees to think seriously, and this was particularly important for women—though actually, at the time, she had addressed her remarks to a male trainee.

When I asked Li Ann what she most enjoyed about her work, she said without any hesitation: "The people. After working so long, work is just *part* of the job. People element [gives] some motivation—and in other departments [of the hospital]. Helping people—trainees, not just patients, attendants—all people. To me there is no division. But no division sometimes also no good."

I have described three members of staff with a particularly ethical and sociable stance in their working life. For these women, as with the nurses in Singapore described by Megha Amrith (2013), religious and ethical attitudes, combined with a willingness to engage socially with patients and colleagues, strongly inflected their working lives and relations. It is certainly not coincidental that these staff members were women—this reflects the quite strongly gendered aspects of sociality and working relations in the labs that I described in chapter 2. Of course, many other staff in the lab—both men and women—were less sociable, concentrating more exclusively on their work tasks and maintaining stronger boundaries between work and social matters. But there is no doubt that having some women in the lab like Anne, Kamariah, and Li Ann, for whom the relationships of the lab were of great importance, affected the quality of the working environment for everyone. Male managers often capitalized on these propensities by using them to smooth over difficulties, ensuring good working relations and the productivity of the labs. The "domesticating" effects of their sociability thus spread beyond their own particular workbench or section.

Laboratory Knowledge

One of the ways in which I tried to understand how connections might be made between life in the lab and life outside was to ask lab workers whether they ever applied their technical knowledge in contexts outside work. Many members of the labs staff told me about giving advice to friends and relatives on blood tests and the results of tests. This might involve explaining to parents or other relatives about the nature of particular tests they were required to have or interpreting results, or it might be on other health matters less directly connected with their own work. Sometimes they would advise on which doctor it would be best to see at the hospital; sometimes they might explain a medical condition or a course of treatment or diet change recommended by a doctor to a friend or relative. This kind of advice giving was a normal part of the background to their work; it went alongside performing diagnostic tests in the labs on samples that might originate in patients with whom they were familiar.

Often lab staff smoothed the path of a friend or relative as they were going through the hospital by helping to make sure they didn't have to wait for too long. In the same way, they talked to each other about their own medical concerns, or those of their relatives, discussing various possible courses of action and different treatments. Thus, in my interview with Anne quoted above, she mentioned how she realized that her mother had a kidney problem and that this kind of thing was one source of connection between her home and working life. Requests for help or advice could of course also be a source of irritation. Many people in the lab complained about having to give advice to their relatives. One medical lab technologist told me, "[They] always think we're doctors, ask us questions as if we know everything. My neighbors always ask me to buy urine catheters. Otherwise, neighbor asks me to buy Panadol—hospital Panadol, he says, very good." She found this amusing because in fact the lab staff did join together to buy over-the-counter remedies in bulk, with each person taking one or two bottles, but because the hospital drugs were more expensive, they were not ordered through the hospital.

It was not all that surprising to find that expertise in health matters was a source of requests for information and advice from friends and relatives of those who worked in the clinical pathology labs, and I could give many examples of this kind of flow of information from the lab. But it was also relatively easy to track different kinds of knowledge about health matters flowing in the opposite direction—into the lab. I have already mentioned that MLTs and other staff talked about illnesses and possible cures in terms of Chinese, Ayurvedic, and Malay medical knowledge and practices. An openness to various different kinds of medical knowledge and practice that are generally available in Malaysia characterized discussions about health and illness in the lab. And members of staff from different ethnic backgrounds were interested in the similarities and differences between various medical traditions. For some, however, their involvement in these medical traditions went further than this. One trainee in the lab told me he had learned about Ayurvedic and Chinese medicine on his university course but his grandfather had also been an Ayurvedic healer, and his mother and father had carried on this tradition but from books. Traditional Chinese and Indian medicine, he said, were quite close. These systems relied on an idea of balance:

> Cold and warm, yin and yang—about balance. Whereas here [he gestured round the lab], it is based on symptoms. Current drugs—cure is temporary only. TCM [traditional Chinese medicine] and Indian medicine look at whole body. Drugs have side effects. TCM has less side effects. Based on forefathers, and on experience.

Several of the medical lab technologists I got to know had a more sustained engagement with Chinese medicine, which in two cases involved their fathers—though in different ways. One, Yew Shan, had worked as a medical lab technologist for six years. Her father ran a Chinese medicine shop near a local market that had been established by her grandfather. Yew Shan was a conduit of information about Chinese medicine in the lab. She told me that her parents worked long hours in their shop, from 7:30 in the morning to 10:00 at night. Now that her parents were old, she and her sisters were concerned about the hours their father worked and were trying to find a way to help him. She told me her father had originally wanted her to study pharmacy so that the shop could be half a pharmacy and half a Chinese medicine shop, but she hadn't gotten the necessary grades. Now Yew Shan was trying to help her younger sister find out about studying Chinese medicine so that the latter might take over the shop, but she also sometimes talked about working there herself.

Another medical lab technologist, Kar Yin, with a degree in genetics and molecular biology, had worked in the lab for five years and, when I spoke to her in 2008, had for some years also been training for three nights a week to be a practitioner of Chinese medicine at a clinic in George Town. I asked her how she had gotten interested in Chinese medicine. She told me it was because her father had a stroke when she was in high school: "[He] couldn't walk. Was admitted to GH [General Hospital]. Couldn't do anything. Then went to get acupuncture . . . [she showed me where the needles were inserted]—and could walk. Miracle. Another one [patient] couldn't talk. Needle in [his] tongue—could count one to ten." Kar Yin also told me that she herself only took herbal medicine rather than Western medicine and had never taken antibiotics. She said she couldn't swallow pills and that she wanted to strengthen her immune system against infection. Some days after this conversation, Kar Yin told me that she'd like to work fully as a Chinese medicine practitioner in the future. I enquired whether she thought her scientific training would be useful. She said it would: "Maybe teaches logical thinking."

In many ways it is hardly surprising to find Chinese, Malay, or Ayurvedic medical knowledge having a presence in the lab since all of these are widespread in most contemporary urban contexts in Malaysia. But I was intrigued by the way medical lab technologists moved between different systems of medical knowledge. On a visit to the labs in 2012, Kar Yin was happy to explain more about the basis of the postpartum restrictions that I described earlier. She told me that "heaty" food (which endows the body with heat, a classification from traditional Chinese medicine that also has a correspondence with Malay humoral ideas) seals the pores of the skin so that wind can't enter and subsequently cause problems to the bones.

Heaty food also for blood; [women] take special medicine to replenish blood. After childbirth both wind and blood are important but wind more important—because pores are everywhere. Women after child-birth are weak, therefore eat heaty foods to get energy. Energy and blood loss makes you weak. Sesame oil and ginger are heaty. Ginger is good for circulation.

I asked her about replenishing the blood, and she told me that Chinese dates, red meat, and red beans are good for this and that, as in Malay articulations, food becomes blood in Chinese medical ideas. I went on to inquire whether bloodletting was good in cases where the body is "heaty," and she said, "Yes, a little bit"—for stroke patients and for fevers. She explained that the fingertips, ears, and neck are acupuncture points. "For stroke patients, just one or two drops of thick, dark blood [are taken] to help reduce blood clot going to brain—before going to hospital." This, she explained, "lets go [i.e., releases the] bad energy—*iechi*. When the outer layer gets sick, this shouldn't be allowed to go in deeper to inner layer, third layer."[4]

I asked Kar Yin whether she treated her colleagues, and she told me she did—for example, squeezing one or two drops of blood from the right side of the left thumb and the left side of the right thumb. She had tried this for one of her colleagues when he had a sore throat, and it had helped. Chinese medicine, she told me, aims to cure the symptoms, not the disease. "Every patient is different—not generalizable"—unlike Western medicine. And, she explained, a patient's symptoms change as the disease progresses. Symptoms are part of the whole process of a disease—so Chinese doctors tell patients to return after a few days to see whether they are cured or getting worse. She said the "principles of diagnosing in Chinese medicine are feel, smell, touch, and ask, in order to diagnose. Feel pulse—three fingers for different symptoms, on different wrists; feel whether hot. Some for inner and some for outer layer of body."

Crucially, rather than attempting to isolate her background in Chinese medicine from her lab work, Kar Yin told me that it was good to share knowledge. Here the circulation of expertise and knowledge, like that of food or ethical concern, can be seen as a form of sociality. Many of her lab colleagues come to her for advice, Kar Yin said, but she doesn't charge for this. It "helps me remember too. Should share knowledge." When I asked her whether it wasn't confusing operating in different systems, Kar Yin said, "It used to be confusing; not anymore." The "lab system to diagnose;

Chinese medicine for cure." In the end, she said, it was "not bad to work in hospital—can compare alternatives. See more than others; know both systems—more choices." Rather than excluding each other, here different systems of medical knowledge apparently increase the available alternatives for treatment. And this reinforces the suggestion that the separations underlying laboratory practices are unstable and porous.

Uncanny Presences

I began this chapter with stories about ghostly appearances and the suggestion that uncertainty about the presence of ghosts in the labs and blood banks was the subject of considerable interest. Because of their association with death, it is widely acknowledged that hospitals are places where ghosts are liable to appear. Since blood is well known to attract spirits in Malaysia, it seemed obvious to attempt to follow these ghostly leads to the blood banks and labs. But, as I discovered, such matters were not straightforward. To understand the significance of their disputed presence, I have found suggestive Freud's ([1919] 2003) emphasis on the link between the uncanny (*unheimlich*) and what was once well known or familiar.

During one discussion about whether ghosts might be present in the labs or blood banks, one of the medical lab technologists, Shanthi, stated that it wasn't safe for the hospital to let staff work alone in these spaces. Another agreed, adding that the ghosts didn't show up on the security cameras. Shanthi mentioned that she, like some of the others, had heard about strange knockings on ward doors. When the nurses tried to get out of the room, she said, they found the door has been locked from the outside. Her colleague confirmed this, noting that the room in question was the one that had previously been the lab's on-call rest room: "Luckily don't use it." It was generally agreed that, although nurses see a lot of ghosts, they aren't themselves subject to their attacks because of their white uniforms. One of the other medical lab technologists mentioned that there were no ghosts in the nursing college itself because there were no patients there. Another colleague teased Shanthi that she wanted to hear more stories but was also scared by them, confirming my sense that these discussions evoked pleasurable excitement as well as fear.

On the following day, over their breakfast, two of the MLTs, Kamariah and Shanthi, were discussing the story of the nurses who had seen the headless ghost. Kamariah mentioned that "GH [General Hospital] has more ghosts." She said this was "because they have a mortuary there. Sometimes they hold a dead person for three months because no one claims. Here not. Don't accept patients if [their condition is] very serious, or without deposit from family. Just have holding area for corpses—one day to claim." Agreeing, Shanthi then mentioned that she was due to be on call the next day, but she was scared to be alone.

Running through the conversations, we can discern a diagnostic of different spaces (in marked counterpoint to that governing the consumption of food)—with certain locations being apparently more prone to attract ghosts. Everyone seemed to agree that hospital wards and the old labs— which had been on the ground floor, exposed to the outside, near the hospital drains, and therefore dirty—were known for such events.[5] Others, not frequented by patients—like the nursing college—were not. Abandoned wards, locked rooms, the morgue, and, even more macabre, the "psychy ward toilets" were likely venues for ghosts.

Stories circulated not only through the spaces of each hospital but also between them. It was perhaps not surprising, then, to be told that the mortuary of the General Hospital was a gathering point for ghosts. In another hospital's labs, one of the more senior medical lab technologists told me that he too had heard from one of the maintenance engineers of a medical technology company about the ghosts in other hospital labs. There weren't any in the labs where he worked, Sam said, because these were located in a separate building from the hospital. But of course, he added, the main hospital itself was a different matter. Sam went on to inquire about the working relations between colleagues in the other set of labs—as if sensing that there might be some connection between the quality of these and uncanny occurrences. His colleagues, however, did not seem quite so certain of the security of their own workspaces. One told me that their lab did get ghosts even though it was housed in a separate building: "Lab is still in hospital compound." She told me that she was scared in the compound at night: "First thing we should be afraid of is thieves. Second thing is ghosts." Another medical lab technologist said she wasn't frightened: "On wards, wear uniform—ghosts don't bother [us]—they know [we're] working to save lives." The connection between thieves and ghosts here is not coincidental, and we have already encountered it in the newspaper accounts of the "public life of blood." There I referred to James Siegel's (1998) suggestion that amid the social dislocations experienced in New Order Indonesia under Suharto, new types of criminals emerged and replaced more familiar kinds of haunting caused by ghosts. While ghost stories were told "with amusement and satisfaction," newspaper stories of such new criminal types spoke of "trauma and shock" (Siegel 1998, 100).

On another occasion, a medical lab technologist told a story about the mother of a friend of hers who had been a patient giving birth in the hospital and had been disturbed by ghosts at night in her room. She related how a nurse had come to the room and fainted. Her friend's mother just pretended it was normal, she said, although she could actually see the ghost, and pressed the alarm to get help for the nurse. A colleague listening to her story then asked whether ghosts were also attracted to the blood bank. "No," she said, "that's OK because the blood is all in containers. It's spilled blood, or the blood of childbirth, that's not OK." In her account of popular religion in Penang, Jean DeBernardi notes the impurity of menstrual blood and the blood of childbirth: "The Hokkien term that describes ritual impurity (*lasam*) also names ghosts and female sexual fluids, both of which are regarded as dirty" (DeBernardi 2006, 124). She recounts the case of a woman who entered a temple during the period of postnatal confinement. Because of this she was unlucky and saw a ghost as she fell asleep and then became ill (107–8).

Stories in the labs are permeated with various kinds of evaluation—the likelihood of ghosts appearing correlates, as we have seen, with the different uses of space in the present and past as well as with the kinds of people who frequent it, and with concerns about practices of containment of blood. Patients who are near death attract ghosts, as do spaces associated with death. The pervasive risks of the workspaces of the hospital and the labs, which were noted in chapter 3, are registered here in the idiom of the uncanny. The use of the English term "ghosts" avoided any specificity about the ethnic association or particular type or name of spirits involved, but it depicted them in vaguer terms as an unexplained touch or presence and thus fitted the multiethnic character of these urban hospitals.[6] The inability to name the ghostly presences of the lab, like the uncertainty about whether they had actually penetrated the boundaries of the labs or not, captures the myriad and uncertain dangers of these spaces and their often unattributed but pervasive risks.

But although ghosts and spirit encounters are associated with fear, stories about ghosts in the labs are told with considerable relish—as is more generally the case in Malaysia and as we saw in the newspaper accounts cited earlier. Thus their antics, like those described for Vietnam by Heonik Kwon (2008), have an entertaining aspect. One could see this as both relieving the tedium of everyday work and evoking its strange terrors in a known and paradoxically "homely" register. As Laura Bear (2007) has suggested, ghosts are certainly uncanny, but they also allow the translation of unknown risks and dangers into a language that springs from home and domestic life (Freud [1919] 2003).

Of course, another side of risk is trust, and the medical lab technologists I knew were well aware that their safety was a matter not only of hospital management policies, or of their own work practices, but also of those of their colleagues. During a training session for a newly installed blood grouping machine in one of the labs that I revisited in 2012, a biotech company rep was running through frequently encountered problems. As he was going through the start-up procedures for the machine, he mentioned that each member of staff should have their own password with which to log on in case a problem arose later, "to rule yourself out," as he put it. One of the lab staff explained in response that, once it was set up and running for the day, different members of staff did not usually log on separately. The biotech rep pointed out the disadvantages of this practice in terms of exposing staff to possible blame for the mistakes of their colleagues. No one spelled out the equally plausible scenario (or risk) that blame for an error might thereby be clearly attributable to oneself. Meeting a marked lack of response, the rep tailed off rather lamely, "Oh, so you trust your colleagues," and reiterated that the company recommended each worker having their own password.

I was often asked by staff in one set of labs about the working practices, spaces, and social relations in the other labs in which I had spent time, and I was struck by how interested those I talked to were in what I might know about how matters stood in other hospitals. It also seemed hard to avoid a connection between the more frequent ghostly appearances and discussions in one lab and the more difficult and sometimes tense relations that existed between colleagues there. In one set of labs, staff seemed to work particularly well as a team. In another, things were more complex, and some relations seemed strained. It was perhaps not coincidental that in the latter working environment I encountered several cases of illness among staff, as well as considerable anxiety about dangers associated with the workplace, including risks of infection, worries about fumigation systems that might not be working effectively, accidents, and the long-term hazards of working with chemical reagents. Explicitly or not, a connection between strained relations between colleagues and the presence of ghosts was indicated too in some of the questions I was asked by those who worked in other hospitals. It was clear that different people had different opinions about the likelihood of encountering ghosts; these were matters for discussion and speculation. And it became apparent that some people were more likely to have such experiences than others. When I began asking about ghosts in the labs, I was told that I should speak to a particular medical lab technologist who had had many such experiences. When I talked to him, Thomas said,

> Only in old lab. Hear sounds going on; hear footsteps. Feel like something eerie; cold on head. Turned around and see nothing. One incident, I thought I saw something sitting in [the lab manager's] old office. Turned around, not there. [I] think they're everywhere. Just where and when manifest is different.

But, as in Sharon's account with which I began this chapter, any certainty about the new space of the lab seemed somehow provisional: "Sometimes still get feeling in this lab. In bewitching hour—3:00 a.m. or something. Some people more sensitive. In old lab heard similar stories. Here in new lab haven't heard any yet."

These comments strongly suggested that the ghostly presences of the hospital might be only temporarily—or just—kept at bay outside the blood bank and clinical pathology labs. While some of the staff seemed pretty sure that, as long as these spaces were unfrequented by patients and blood was kept in sealed containers, their boundaries would be secure, for others these matters were uncertain. If ghosts had not yet been encountered, this did not mean that there was no chance they would be in the future.

Animation

Obvious questions that arose in relation to the uncertain presence of ghosts in the labs were what exactly they might be attracted by and whether something about these spaces made them particularly prone to hauntings. The answers were quite variable. Some said that, since they were "handling blood," it was "not surprising." Others maintained that blood stored in sealed bags or containers was not a problem and that the labs were actually not particularly prone to such haunting. It was spilled blood that might cause ghosts to come. Still others told me that sites that were especially dirty or smelly attracted ghosts: "It's the hospital: bad spirits attracted by bad smell of blood maybe—and dirt." And here we might draw a connection to concerns that were often articulated about keeping the labs clean and tidy, not leaving open samples around, avoiding spillages, making sure centrifuges and other equipment had been properly cleaned of traces of blood each day. All of these were regarded as part of the proper running of the clinical pathology labs and important for the health and safety of those who worked there. Without negating the importance of these functions, it is possible to surmise that neglecting such tasks might contribute to the presence of the uncanny in the labs.

The ambiguous presence of ghosts thus provided a repertoire for articulating the strangeness and pollution of the lab spaces. It also suggested further questions about how the lab staff regarded the blood samples and donations that were so much a part of their everyday working lives. In particular, I was led to wonder about the vitality of blood. While questions about this drew a blank with some of the medical lab technologists, others held interestingly varied views. Some gave what seemed intended as a "scientific" answer to my questions about whether they thought blood was alive, saying that, during the time donated blood was kept in packs to be used for transfusion, it was alive but only for a limited time—depending on the kind of bag and the preservative and nutrient used. For whole blood this would be thirty-five or forty-two days. Most said that blood samples in test tubes were not alive, or not really alive, or only alive for a few days. Others mentioned more arbitrary time lengths, saying for example, "blood when taken is alive—maybe for 12 hours or so," but emphasized that this was their

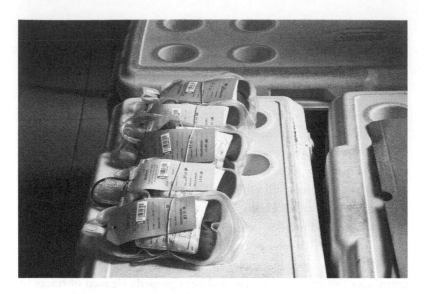

Labeled blood is ready for transfusion in sealed bags.

own opinion. Others were less sure, or said they didn't think that blood was a living thing. Some referred explicitly to the life-giving properties of donated blood, saying, "When in packs, yes; in packs can save lives." One medical lab technologist carefully specified, "Blood *was* alive; once taken, in stasis—like cryo; then [when it's] put in body, comes alive."

These answers suggest considerable ambiguity as well as uncertainty about blood's animated qualities. And, for some staff, the question related directly to the separations that they understood to be a requirement for their work. When I asked one senior medical lab technologist whether she thought blood was alive, she told me, "Inside lab, I differentiate. I try not to think about it—sample tubes, bags—can't do work otherwise. But outside, yes." As the senior medical lab technologist went off to get some samples, I turned to the trainee working beside her and repeated my question. "It is alive," she said without hesitation. "Can tell you many things—key to mystery." "What mystery?" I asked. "Human mystery," came her reply.

We saw in chapter 3 that the separations of lab work were explained as learned through training, but clearly there was still scope for elisions and slippages in what blood stands for or how it is understood. Sometimes these were revealed not simply in the answers to my questions but in the connections made to other topics. Thus when I asked one senior member of the lab staff if she thought blood was alive, she replied, "Not really alive." And then, immediately and unprompted, she followed this up: "Hospital is dirty place—a lot of mess, a lot of suffering. That's why got a lot of spirits—all hospitals. Here the cardiac ward—got a lot of suffering, and pediatric ward—spirits of children calling." Here the living qualities of blood are denied—but seemingly only to be evoked in the idiom of spirits called forth by mess, dirt, death, and suffering.

Such discussions give a strong sense of the ambiguities of blood and of the workspaces of the labs. Some lab staff members told me blood was alive, some said it was not. For some, blood's animation is associated with the world outside the lab, with people, mess, and spirits; and a separation between these worlds must be actively maintained. Others, however, asserted blood's living qualities in the very terms of scientific knowledge, invoking expiration dates and the transfusible capacities of blood. Bridging these different kinds of knowledge and different worlds is the idea of a mystery—the notion, articulated to me by many who worked in the labs, that not only is blood the most revealing of all bodily samples in diagnostic terms, but also that it may hold the answer to questions of illness and suffering, life and death.

Conclusion

I began this chapter with tales about ghosts that might possibly have breached the boundary of the labs. Ghosts, food, fishponds, relatedness, religion and ethics, scuba diving, childbirth, Chinese, Malay, and Ayurvedic medicine—the story so far has involved some improbable juxtapositions. As Emily Martin has written, the "space in which science and culture are co-constituted is discontinuous, fractured, convoluted, and in constant change. To traverse such a space, we need an image of process that allows strange bedfellows, odd combinations, and discontinuous junctures" (1998, 36). Behind all this is the routine work of the lab that I described in chapter 3. This is highly technical work, and the medical lab technologists are under strong pressure from the hospital management—enforced through rigorous regimens of standard operating procedures, protocols, and monitoring—to constantly improve the speed, standards, and accuracy of their results.

I have suggested that—like food but in a markedly different register—traces of dangerous, transgressive, and uncanny presences can be seen as a kind of moral barometer both of the pervasive risks of these workspaces and of the social relations within them, and that they indicate the fragile status of the boundaries of the labs and blood banks. Although members of the public have only restricted access to these spaces, and they are apparently well-ordered, high-tech, and ultramodern working environments, we have seen how other nonwork kinds of sociality, which have their basis in kinship connections as well as religious and ethical commitments, also leave their mark. The dangerous sense of the uncanny suggests that the domestication of the workspace may be seen as an ambivalent process. Boundaries between the labs and the outside world of the hospital might, after all, not be secure; the presence of death in the hospital might invade the labs; familiar forms of sociality between colleagues might break down. Work protocols and regulatory regimens cannot completely guarantee the health or safety of medical lab technologists—however meticulously they are implemented. The safety and familiarity of these zones is at best imperfect and provisional. Those who work in these spaces can perhaps all too easily imagine that morally calibrated social connections and their penumbra of memory, apprehended as the threatening presence of ghosts, might take precedence over the routine technological processes of the labs and blood banks.

The stories I have told about life in the lab may seem inconsequential; they concern matters that are sometimes fleeting or peripheral to the main work processes. I have highlighted the visible and strong effort made by staff to domesticate the working environment and to make it a sociable space. Li Ann's comment that "work is just *part* of the job" is at the heart of this story. But why should this matter? What are the implications of the "uneven seepage" (Rapp 1999, 303) between the world of everyday sociality, kinship, and life in the lab? The depiction I have given of those who work in the labs and blood banks might appear simply to echo other ethnographies of the workplace that depict permeable boundaries between work and other aspects of life (see, for example, Mollona 2005; Yanagisako 2002). But my argument has two further strands that are more specific to the context described here: one has to do with risk, and the other with translatability—I take the latter first.

The idioms of shared knowledge and sociality depicted in this chapter—expertise in different medical systems, commensal patterns, kinship, ethics, discussions about ghosts—are strikingly interethnic. All of these idioms can be attached in Malaysia to ethnically particular practices. They thus have the capacity to coalesce or resolve themselves along familiar ethnic lines. But what is important here is that, in this ethnically plural, urban, technologically advanced, Malaysian working environment, where many of the workers are young or in early middle age, ideas and practices of sociality, which might formerly have been (or even in the present might be) ethnically specific, are to a very considerable degree translatable. In chapter 2 I suggested that these workspaces are the sites of an emerging shared urban Malaysian culture, which, although it carries the potential to divide along ethnic lines, is in many respects ethnically plural. Resting on knowledge and familiarity that cross ethnic boundaries, it has the capacity to contribute to more general and abstract notions of Malaysian citizenship that, like other recent and more political developments, and like blood donation (see chapter 1), transcend ethnic lines.[7] Of course, the potential for food proscriptions, marriage, or medical practices, which are often considered constitutive of ethnicity, to be translatable or shared across ethnic boundaries also carries potentially worrying connotations. New forms of sociality may have the potential to undermine old certainties about identity and affiliation. They thus also carry risks, and we have seen that, because of the nature of the work carried out in them, the labs are in any case risky spaces.

I have described how the processes of domestication considered in this chapter render a strikingly unfamiliar world more familiar. For all their appearance of well-ordered laboratory efficiency, however, there is no disguising the fact that these workspaces are also hazardous, and this is clearly recognized by those who work there. Well-maintained boundaries between different spatial zones, standard operating procedures, safety protocols, and a concern with hygiene cannot, after all, guarantee the health and safety of those who work in these spaces. Whether from a needle prick injury, infectious microbes, or chemical reagents, these personnel know all too well that their health can easily be put at risk—and this was underlined, as we saw in chapter 3, by the manner in which they spoke of the potential dangers of their work. Beyond their own health, they are also aware of the potentially devastating consequences that mistakes in their work could have for the health of others. The effects of a diagnostic test misread or carelessly carried out, blood that has not been properly cross-matched for transfusion, or donated blood inadequately screened—the list of potential errors and their spiraling consequences is endless. The implications of the dangers of these workplaces thus extend well beyond the local context. The history of contaminated blood scandals in France, the UK, and China, among other places, demonstrates that the stakes may be very high indeed (Feldman and Bayer 1999; Shao 2006; Shao and Scoggin 2009; Starr 1998). It should be emphasized here that the regulatory systems in which Malaysian hospitals participate are both local and international. Members of the lab staff were continually reminded of the importance of accuracy and carefulness in their work by managers, and the regulatory practices of the labs and hospitals involved the routine collection and display of statistics to support this.

An emphasis on the sociality of the workspace undoubtedly renders it more enjoyably habitable and reduces the negative effects of pressures to increase productivity or the sense of dangers just kept at bay. In chapter 3, I suggested that "rehumanizing" samples and forms has a positive effect on ensuring the engagement of medical lab technologists with their work, and thus enhances its quality. But, from another point of view, the obligations of friendship and kinship might, paradoxically, be understood to have the opposite effect. It is not hard to imagine conflicts of interest over the reporting of the infectious illnesses of colleagues or mistakes in procedures. Sociability can simultaneously make the world of the lab seem safe and potentially undermine regulatory regimes or standard operating procedures—and thus contribute to risky work conditions. This suggests that, far from being inexplicable, the uncertain and threatening presence of the uncanny expresses the ambivalence and provisionality of processes of domestication in these spaces. A "shadowy residue" left by the work of domestication captures just this sense of implicit danger. In this light, the overdetermined interest in whether ghosts might or might not invade the

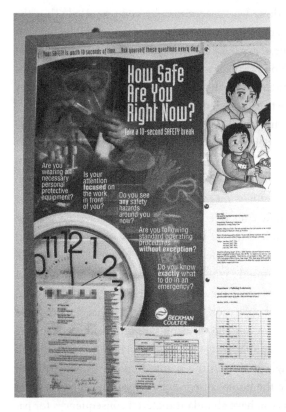

A poster warns about
safety in the workplace.

labs makes clear that domestication cannot fully dissolve the risks associated with this kind of work.

Significantly, it has long been recognized that the entanglements of *commercial* interest might potentially undermine the safety of blood services. That the safety of donated blood rests on the disinterestedness of voluntarily donated gifts was exactly Richard Titmuss's ([1970] 1997) point (see also Rabinow 1999; Tutton 2002).[8] This concern connects directly to the issues discussed here; it is not only commercial interests, however, but also ethical and social obligations that might conceivably compromise the safety of blood. Tellingly, Titmuss's argument dovetails neatly with that of Latour (1993) about the importance of the work of "purification" to perceptions of the validity of scientific endeavors. If the gift might not be disinterested, or if the work of purification is only a mask, then the modern, scientifically valid, safe products of these workspaces may be compromised. Thus the creation of an insulated, disinterested world in the labs and blood banks is apparently the guarantee of accuracy and safety as well as the availability of an adequate supply of blood to meet transfusion needs; it also ensures public trust. Slippages are potential break points in perceptions about reliability that may undermine the trust of patients and publics.

The separation of the lab from the world outside, and the many microprocesses of separation that are integral to the work of the lab, is always precarious. Such divisions are unstable, just as the samples that medical lab technologists encounter are also unstable entities (Singleton 1998). And this is partly because they are maintained by people who, as I have shown, are themselves fully embedded in nexuses of relations and situated simultaneously in multiple different social locations within and beyond the lab. The domestication I have described here, rather than being one side of a binary that is opposed to the work processes of the labs, is in fact embedded in them. It is because the consequences of incomplete separations, or entanglements of obligation, may be literally lethal, and may pile into each other, that doctors and blood bank staff are concerned, as they often told me, about their public image. Mistakes have the capacity to feed quickly and devastatingly back into the many domains in which blood participates—including the bodies of patients. Lapses in the procedures of labs and blood banks can have abundant material consequences for patients and simultaneously have extraordinary ideological propulsion to penetrate many realms of moral discourse, implicating trust in health care and public safety and ultimately in political regimes. In this sense, the projection of such slippages onto the external, dangerous, but simultaneously familiar agency of ghosts may, as Laura Bear (2007) suggests, paradoxically provide a certain kind of reassurance. In an ideal world (one in which the national and international regulatory regimens governing the procedures carried out in blood banks and clinical pathology labs are perfectly effective), the entanglements of kinship, "culture," and human interest would be banished from the spaces of the lab. But work cannot proceed in a such a vacuum.

These ghostly presences that are only provisionally kept at bay outside the blood bank and clinical pathology labs speak of the fragile status of the boundaries of the lab and also of how much might be at stake. When Li

Ann told me that "work is just *part* of the job" she immediately followed this with a qualification: "no division sometimes also no good." The porous seepage between work and social life, between the up-to-date, technologized labs and the world outside—with its inescapable social obligations and haunting memories—is intrinsic to the way life is carried on in the clinical pathology labs and blood banks. But such seepages also have the potential to disrupt work undertaken in these spaces—and lives lived far beyond them.

CONCLUSION

What separates the living from the dead? · Life's presence is manifest to
the senses, yet ever eludes the reach of our comprehension. We plainly see the
metamorphoses of vitality in someone running, stopping, looking back, turning pale; we can hear the supple force of life in the sharpness of precise dic-
tion, and in the soft insinuations of tone; we can even grasp vital power with
our fingers, here at the wrist, feel it pulsating or flowing. But in the end the
mystery persists.

—KURIYAMA, *The Expressiveness of the Body*

Tracing the social life of blood in Penang has taken us on some unexpected
pathways and highlighted some improbable juxtapositions. It is time to gather
up these threads and to consider their implications. What does blood signify
for the people depicted in this book? We have encountered a patient undergoing heart surgery whose animatory state is impossible to know. We have met
blood donors whose donations, recorded in donor booklets, seem to encapsulate the history of their lives and are a memorial to kinship connections;
a donor for whom the significance of donation has apparently expanded to
substitute for such connections; and another who quips that his booklet, the
material record of his ethical actions, might be a "passport to heaven." We have
seen blood bagged and tagged in the labs, screened and cross-matched for
transfusion, sealed in labeled Vacutainers, test tubes, and blood packs, but
seemingly reluctant to shed its traces of personal and social connection, its
resonances of kinship, gender, ethnicity, illness, memory, and hope.

In the apparently sealed and sanitized spaces of the labs, we have found
a dense social connectivity with crisscrossing networks of commensal
relations that are enacted in hospital cafeterias and local eateries, including

global chains such as KFC, but which also involve food grown or cooked at home. This commensality produces, expresses, and reflects an archaeology of relations based in friendship, kinship, and marriage that stretches within and beyond the labs and the hospitals in which they are situated. The fishponds of the labs express containment and control and require the cooperative engagement of those who maintain them. They are an aesthetic form expressive of a nonbinary domesticity, combining work and play, functionality and decoration, the wild and the tame, home and public institution. We have seen how joking, banter, stories of family life, and ghostly tales are part of collegial relations, as is the capacity to draw the technology of the labs into social networks. Curiosity, social engagement, and ethical and religious dispositions shape and inform how people perform the mundane and routinized work of the labs. Entanglements among work, personal histories, and social life, rather than compromising lab safety and procedures, enhance the quality of work and the results obtained. Processes of domestication and rehumanization, far from being incidental, have been shown to be integral to the work of the labs.

In the introduction to this book I set out two complementary lines of inquiry: the first was to show how an ethnography of blood work in Penang might illuminate wider social processes in Malaysia; the second was, through that ethnography, to explore more broadly what kind of thing blood is and how we can account for its special qualities. Beyond these two strands of discussion, and linking them together, we can detect a third question underlying this work: What does the depiction of these particular Malaysian worlds reveal more generally about lives lived in modernity?

Following the routes along which blood travels in specific biomedical settings, I suggested, might bring contemporary Malaysia into focus in a new way. The urban spaces of the clinical pathology labs and blood banks, and the people encountered there, might afford an unexpected lens through which to understand wider social processes in Penang. Placing ethnic, religious, or kinship ties in the background, in multiethnic, urban, highly technologized work spaces, where religion or kinship are of no necessary or predictable relevance, has allowed us to see how thoroughly they permeate the seemingly enclosed and hypermodern environment of the lab.

McKinnon and Cannell's (2013) emphasis on the significant presence of kinship within the institutions of modernity, which runs counter to the myths we tell ourselves about the fundamental distinction between "traditional" and "modern" worlds, has been amply borne out here. Rather than being a realm from which kinship has been excised, we find the moral and emotional traces of kinship and relatedness widely dispersed in these seemingly hypermodern and highly technologized workplaces. Histories of connection are enfolded into the motivations of blood donors, relations between colleagues in the labs, everyday dealings between lab staff and patients, and the lab staff's daily encounters with bodily samples and transfusion packs. While the work of the labs proceeds through the enactment of separations between these spaces and the outside world, the relational qualities of samples, patients, donors, and staff supersede such acts of boundary-making.

Attending to public discourses about blood reinforces these insights. The apparently iconic blood sample of the leader of Malaysia's opposition, Anwar Ibrahim, seemed to encapsulate the political moment of 2008 and its unexpected possibilities. Representing, for some, the corrupt practices of the established political elite anxious to hold on to power, and, for others, the possibly nefarious doings of a charismatic and unpredictable opposition leader, Anwar's blood sample was an object of considerable contestation. Through a process of scientific testing, possibly undertaken by "foreign experts," some maintained that this blood sample had the capacity to "reveal the truth." But behind such improbable assertions one could discern a complex and uneasy conjuncture of discourses about science and modernity, as well as a rich archaeology of ideas about the power and meanings of bodily substances, sexual practices, and corrupt political dealings.

• • •

Our journey began with blood donation campaigns and blood banks, where donors are animated by desires to "save a life," memories of past kinship, and the available material and moral recompense for giving blood. These inducements are threaded through individual life stories that take account of histories of employment, residence, and kinship. We have seen how newspaper reports about blood and organ donation, petty crime, and other matters evoke moral evaluations about their protagonists—as is also the case when blood bank staff encounter potential donors. These assessments encompass judgments about sexual behavior, drug use, and kinship, and they also rely on ideas and received stereotypes about gender and ethnicity. The entanglements of "race," religion, and moral worth in newspaper reports, at blood campaigns, on donor forms, and in the blood banks and labs are perhaps one particularly Malaysian aspect of the stories that I have told. As we saw in chapter 2, such matters also affect the life chances and educational opportunities of Malaysian citizens—including those who become lab technicians or medical lab technologists—in direct and material ways.

The world of the clinical pathology labs and blood banks is closed to most outsiders. As the doors to these departments proclaim, unauthorized visitors are not allowed. But inside these chilly, quiet, and well-ordered spaces we have also encountered some unlikely associations. There is, to be sure, the routine work of the labs and blood banks, involving the latest sophisticated diagnostic tools, up-to-date medical technology that enables diagnostic tests on blood, urine, and other samples to take place, and the separation of blood into blood products that can be stored and cross-matched, ready for transfusion. These tasks are carried out by trained medical lab technologists with university degrees in subjects such as biology, genetics, or biochemistry. In this controlled laboratory environment we have also discovered a sociality embedded in the idioms of kinship—relations between siblings, engaged couples, husbands and wives, and parents, babies and children, and friends who have worked alongside each other for many years. We have encountered a variety of nonallopathic medical treatments and staff who are motivated by an ethic of service and by religious ideals side by side with those who simply value the peace and quiet of the labs and an absence of social engagement. Relations between colleagues are enacted through a range of commensal practices that recall other less technocratic environments. We have learned about scuba diving, Chinese medicine, ornamental fishponds, and ghosts. The lives and concerns of medical lab technologists, their "histories in person" (Holland and Lave 2001), have proved to be neither predictable nor easily circumscribed.

Ethnicity and gender, in their particular Malaysian forms and with their particular Malaysian history, reach into many aspects of the social life of blood—from the forms that blood donors complete to the career opportunities of lab staff and the qualities ascribed to samples, donations, and patients. While we might see these as lending a weight of overdetermined ascriptions to persons, bodily substances, and acts, we have also seen that there is risk, uncertainty, and pleasure associated with working in these multiethnic and highly technologized urban spaces. Commensal and postnatal practices are associated with ethnic and religious differences, but they also, tantalizingly, suggest translatability—the idea that sociality might overcome these barriers. Such a denial of difference might, however, be far more risky, and potentially more world-shattering, than the maintenance of boundaries.

One striking feature of the ethnography that I have presented is the "layeredness" or density of connections that we have been able to trace as blood circulates between different domains. Moving between the bodies of donors or patients and sealed blood bags or Vacutainers, via the labs and blood banks and then, through the interceptions of staff in these locations, back to the same or different patients, blood sheds and acquires different layers of meanings. The connections to the sources of blood in particular donors or patients, as I showed in chapter 3, cannot be severed and are materialized in the labels on samples and bagged blood products. These connections are amplified by staff of the blood banks and labs, who may or may not be familiar with donors or patients when they perform their routine work on samples or on donated blood. Such entanglements are intensified in the wider contexts of public and political discourses about blood and organ donation in Malaysia. We saw in chapter 1 that the blood of donors has both gift- and commodity-like attributes. And because the links between donors and their donated blood, or between samples and their sources in particular patients or donors, are integral to blood bank and lab procedures, the many meanings of blood circulate within the work processes of the lab as well as beyond them. Thus we might speak of the "velocity" or "viscosity" of blood as it flows between different spheres.[1]

Medical lab technologists regard blood as able to reveal the truth about the body in a manner that is unlike other bodily materials, and sometimes, in distinctly nonmodern articulations, they evoke the idea of a "mystery." Blood may seem a less significant donation than a kidney or heart, and its appearance in one among hundreds of similar sample test tubes on a lab bench is hardly spectacular. But the moral qualities of the living persons from which it derives are not easily shed. This perhaps is one lesson we can draw from the contestations over Anwar's blood sample, which embodied in a seemingly overdetermined way not just meanings that I have alluded to here but a whole prehistory of relations among Malaysia's political elite, stretching back at least as far as Mahathir's time as Prime Minister.

The emotional, moral, and truth-revealing qualities of blood evoke potential relational capacities. While blood is not conclusively alive, its uncertain status of animation and its capacity to animate others, as well as the risks of contamination and dangers of infection it carries, are echoed in the uncertain presence of ghosts in the labs. Nor is it coincidental that the question of whether ghosts are attracted by the blood in the labs is a particularly troubling one for those who work there. When doctors and blood bank staff in Penang expressed their concern to me about public perceptions of blood bank practices, including whether patients were charged for blood that had been freely donated, or about "cultural matters" affecting public willingness to donate blood, they were indicating their awareness of how such issues might intrude into the supply of blood available for transfusion. The creation of a wholly insulated, disinterested world in the labs and blood banks, however illusory a prospect, is apparently the guarantee of accuracy and safety as well as the availability of an adequate supply of blood to meet transfusion needs; it thus also ensures public trust. Slippages are potential break points in perceptions about reliability that may undermine the trust of patients and publics.

• • •

Apart from the specificities of Malaysia, I began this book with more general questions about the nature of blood and what its unusual properties signify. Taking what might have turned out to be a rather reductive or literalist turn through blood banks and clinical pathology labs to investigate this question seems not to have led, as we might have expected, to any straightforwardly scientistic or simple materialist conclusions. The ambiguous animation and vitality of blood may be articulated in the idioms of scientific or medical knowledge and also registered in more transcendental terms.

In the introduction I argued that the unusual material qualities of blood are key to its propensity for figurative elaboration. We saw how the dense entanglement of blood's multiple resonances and metaphorical allusions, and their ready familiarity, obscures the effects of this pileup of meanings. Blood would seem to be a paradigmatic case of "multiple naturalization" in Bowker and Star's terms (1999, 312). If it seems a faint hope to be able to observe such processes of naturalization "in action," as it were, the ethnography presented here has been an attempt to show how they occur and to explore their implications.

This ethnography suggests that the quality of animation is at the heart of blood's enlarged capacity for naturalization. On my last day in the labs before leaving Penang in 2012, I asked one of the medical lab technologists who was working in blood chemistry whether blood is alive. After gently reminding me that I had already asked him this question, he responded, "In packs, yes; less in tubes." He continued, "But still in tubes [blood] can tell story of patient's condition. Can then check back to request form to see, and remember. Sometimes still remember [their] face, feel sorry for patient." In this account of work in the labs, which we met in chapter 3, we see how a blood sample in a test tube can tell a patient's story and still carries qualities of a patient's life. This, then, is yet another aspect of blood's vitality.

Referring to the mystery that blood both contains and reveals, medical lab technologists acknowledge its truth-bearing qualities (see Bildhauer 2013; Copeman 2013)—the unique ability it has to disclose what is going on in the bodies of patients—and also its strangely ambiguous status. Blood has an unusual propensity to flow between domains and to overcome boundaries and stoppages between them. It is necessary for life, and transfusion can bring the mortally ill back from the brink, but the question of whether blood is by itself alive has no conclusive answer. Like the artificially stopped heart of a patient undergoing bypass surgery whose vital status is unknowable, with which we began our sanguinary journey, once taken from a donor, blood is in a state of suspended animation. It is "in stasis," ready to come alive or to "save a life."

As the quote from Kuriyama (2002) that appears both in the introduction to this book and at the head of this chapter evocatively captures, there is indeed something mysterious here. Perhaps it should not surprise us then that, if blood may be said to separate the living from the dead, it is also in many cultures understood as the stuff that connects living persons who are related and that distinguishes different kinds of people from each other. This may be elaborated in idioms of kinship, the body, morality, religion, race, and the nation. Already naturalized, blood has the potential to contribute to further naturalizations in many registers of connection and separation. And, as different resonances flow between domains, adhering to and reinforcing each other, they become difficult to disentangle or erase.

The strong association between blood and animation is a general one that is probably elaborated in most, if not all, cultures. Blood's propensity for metaphorization is linked to this association with life itself. And the further tendency for the metaphorical meanings of blood to multiply, and flow with ease across domains that in other contexts are often separated, is linked to the heightened possibility of meanings and references to be naturalized. Understandings transform and loop back on themselves to encompass different versions of older ideas about substances and relationships with multiple temporalities. Blood's aptness for symbolization, I argue, stems from its "animatory power," which predisposes it to accrue metaphorical associations with different temporalities and which themselves have further "naturalizing momentum." These may be general and connected properties of blood, but particular connotations and resonances emerge through locally and culturally specific histories. The contexts investigated in this ethnography reveal the intricate interplay between blood's general and particular meanings. Often it is difficult to say where the general ends and the specific begins, and this of course is part of the very process of naturalization and metaphor.

• • •

In the introduction, I referred to the difficulties Lewis Henry Morgan had with his publishers over his preferred dedication to *Systems of Consanguinity and Affinity of the Human Family*. Thomas Trautmann tells us that when Lewis Henry Morgan first saw the published version of his book on his return from a lengthy trip to Europe in July 1871, "it evoked deep emotions of pride and pain." Morgan wrote in his journal that it "is identified in my mind always with the loss of my dear children, the irreparable calamity of my life." The death of his daughters and the struggle with Joseph Henry over his dedication meant that, for Morgan, the work assumed the "private iconography of a memorial to the dead" (Trautmann 1987, 1). As Morgan understood, even in the most modern and scientific institutions, human life and histories of connection between persons—kinship in the broadest sense—are in fact inseparable.

This reminder of the history of occlusions that is at the heart of the origins of the anthropological study of kinship brings us finally to the question of how this ethnography of blood work in Malaysia speaks to a more general anthropology of people living "modern lives." The entangled figures of blood donors, their booklets, professionals, banterers, items of sophisticated medical technology, protocols of testing and monitoring, forms, fish tanks, labeled blood samples and products, ethical workers, co-diners, food, patients, relatives, and others we have met in this book illustrate the messy complexity of ordinary, everyday life—not just in Malaysia but elsewhere too. The processes of domestication depicted here have a wider resonance than their Malaysian specificity. Their nonbinary embeddedness in the world of the labs reflects the multidimensional character of modern life. The way that blood is handled and contained, overspills its boundaries, and circulates thus speaks to entanglements of everyday experience with which we are all familiar.

A close examination of seemingly routine and understated practices, and the lives of those who enact them, has revealed how the supposedly separate domains of kinship, politics, economics, science, and religion—the hallmark of "modernity"—in fact bleed into each other. In this way the ethnography has taken us beyond the insights of scholars of science and technology studies who have depicted purification, boundary-crossings, instabilities, and multiple objects within laboratory practice. The myth of domaining, as a condition of laboratory life *and* of modernity more generally, has been shown to be just that—a myth. And this is not because laboratory work proceeds in spite of such boundary-crossings but because it *requires* them. Blood work cannot be separated from the sociality of which it is part. If the modes of sociality described here are specifically Malaysian, with particular Malaysian resonances and histories, such entanglement, with all the capacity it generates for the amplification of meaning and for enhancing—or upsetting—experiences of work and other areas of life, goes beyond Malaysia. Seen in this light, blood might not only be the stuff of life but may also hold the key to an anthropology of everyday modern life that captures the intensity of this engagement.

INTRODUCTION

1 Kuriyama shows how the divergent traditions of classical Greek and ancient Chinese medicine both traced vitality to blood and breath (see Kuriyama 2002, 192; see also Francis 2015, 72–73).

2 See Carsten 2011, 2013; Foucault (1978) 1979; Fraser and Valentine 2006; Laqueur 1999.

3 On contemporary expressions of these Chinese notions, see also Adams, Erwin, and Le 2010; Erwin 2006.

4 See, for example, Anagnost 2006; Baud 2011; Chaveau 2011; Erwin 2006; Feldman and Bayer 1999; Laqueur 1999; Rabinow 1999; Shao 2006; Shao and Scoggin 2009; Starr 1998.

5 See Copeman 2009c; Seeman 1999, 2010; Strong 2009; Valentine 2005.

6 See also Adams, Erwin, and Le 2010; Barad 2003; Carsten 2013; Copeman 2013; Hoek 2014; Mumtaz and Levay 2014; Ong 2010b.

7 See also Anidjar 2014, xii; Hoek 2014, 32; Latour 1993; Miller 2005.

8 See Banerjee 2014; Carsten 2013; Copeman 2009b, 2013, 2014; Hoek 2014.

9 Laura Bear's (2014) attentiveness to the heterochrony or multiplicity of modern time as a focus of inquiry and to the layered and sometimes conflicting representations of time it enfolds is pertinent here. Christopher Pinney has posed the question: "What if, instead of assuming that objects and culture are sutured together in national time-space, we start looking for all those objects and images whose evidence appears to be 'deceptive' and whose time does not appear to be 'our' time?" (Pinney 2005, 262–63). Further explorations of the way that nonhuman entities may create temporalities, or participate in their creation—such as those advanced by Georgina Born (2015) for music and Christopher Pinney (2005) for photographic images—seem called for.

10 Newspaper accounts of these events are analyzed more fully in the section preceding chapter 4 (see also Trowell 2015). For an account of Anwar Ibrahim's complex political biography, see Allers 2013.

11 I am not suggesting that bodily matter is the only means by which ties between political rulers and their followers are created or legitimized, or that blood is the only bodily substance that has this kind of symbolic power—bones, for example, are another apparently potent form of bodily matter—as is clear from the discussion of funerary rituals above.

12 For an examination of the importance of "motion," "transportability," or "locomotive sociality" (Bautista 2012a, viii–ix) as a component of the spiritual potency of material objects in plural religious contexts in Southeast Asia, see the essays in Bautista (2012b). A suggestive case from Malaysia is the holy water of the pilgrimage shrine of St. Anne's Church in Bukit Mertajam discussed by Yeoh (2012).

13 On the entanglements of blood, race, kinship, and heredity, see also Foucault (1978) 1979, 147–50; Porqueres i Gené 2007; Stoler 1992, 1997; Wade 1993, 2002, 2007; Williams 1995.

14 For India, see Copeman 2004, 2005, 2008, 2009a, 2009b, 2009c, 2013. On wider south Asia, see Copeman 2014; Simpson 2004, 2009, 2011. For Brazil, see Sanabria 2009; on China, see Adams, Erwin, and Le 2010; on Papua New Guinea, see Street 2009; and for Israel, see Seeman 2010.

15 See Carsten 2013; Copeman 2009b, 2009c; Hugh-Jones 2011. For a discussion of the parallels between blood and organ donation see also Carsten 2011, and for a broader consideration of substance see Carsten 2004; Copeman 2014.

16 See also Banerjee 2014; Hoek 2014, 32.

17 See Anidjar 2014 for a penetrating exploration of blood as "a critique of Christianity." Blood, Anidjar argues, "is the *element* of Christianity, its voluminous mark (citation, context). It is the way in which and upon which Christianity made its mark. More broadly, a consideration of what blood reflects, produces and sustains, what it engenders, must take—as one adopts—the form of a critique of Christianity" (Anidjar 2014, ix, emphasis in original; see also 26). Christianity, for Anidjar, is an exceptional case: "it is for Christianity and for Christianity only that blood becomes a privileged figure for parts and wholes, a figure for a collective of collectives" (2014, 256). The apparent naturalness of blood is produced in Christianity (2014, 256–58). As will be clear, I take in some respects a wider, but also a more ethnographically specific, approach to the question "what is blood?"—one not confined to a particular religion. This should not of course be equated to having a universalist position on the nature of blood.

18 See Lewis 2016, ch. 4; Lubis 2009, 172–73; Roff 1994.

19 See Khoo 1972; Turnbull 2009; Yeoh et al. 2009.

20 See DeBernardi 2004, 84; Mahani Musa 1999; Tan 2009, 14–15.

21 See Bayly and Harper 2005, 2007; Harper 1999.

22 See Hirschmann 1986, 1987; Holst 2012; Manickam 2015, 98–111; Milner 2011; Milner and Ting 2014; Shamsul 1996; Shamsul and Athi 2014.

23 See DeBernardi 2004, ch. 5, for an account of the impact of "ethnic nationalism" on Chinese Malaysians in Penang.

24 The changing relations between the state and Islam in Malaysia, and Islam's increasing importance in legal matters that may affect non-Muslims too, have been discussed by Malaysian social scientists; see, for example, Maznah Mohamad 2010, 2013; Zawawi Ibrahim and Ahmad Fauzi Abdul Hamid 2017.

25 See Brown 2007; Lee 2014; Neville 1998; Selvaratnam 1988.

26 See Carsten 1995a, 1997; Kahn 2006; Milner 2011; E. C. Thompson 2003, 2007.

27 Warner's (2016) brilliant essay traces the connections (among others) between brogues as footwear and speech patterns. She uses the term "brogue" as "a native tongue in the crucial sense that a language is a particular kind of music, not only a sign system on the page or a structure of grammar. It is also a tune, a pattern of sounds and intonation." The sound pattern is in fact what identifies a brogue, Warner argues, and, unlike accents, which denote a second language, they are often characteristic of bilingual or trilingual experience. "You can be at home in a brogue, you can live in it—a sleek and comfortable pair of slippers. . . . A brogue evokes lilt and cadence and pitch and the melodic undulations of speech."

28 Founded in 1971, *The Star* was originally a regional newspaper based in Penang; it went into national circulation in 1976. Under Malaysia's stringent publication laws, its license was revoked in 1987 as part of a government crackdown ("Operation Lalang"), and it was permitted to publish again in 1988. But "since 1988 it has never regained its previous 'liberal flavour'" (Hilley 2001, 120). However, it is sometimes regarded as less closely associated with government than its main English-language rival (with a lower circulation), the *New Straits Times*. *The Star*'s circulation is among the highest in Malaysia at approximately 250,000, with a further 100,000 for its online edition. It is owned by the Malaysian Chinese Association, a political party that is part of the ruling Barisan Nasional coalition (see Hilley 2001, 119–29; https://en.wikipedia.org/wiki/The_Star_(Malaysia), accessed August 5, 2016).

29 See also Gupta, who writes, "Obviously, perceiving them [newspapers] as having a privileged relation to the truth of social life is naive; they have much to offer us, however, when seen as a major discursive form through which daily life is narrativized and collectivities imagined" (1995, 385).

30 See also Bear 2013; Cannell 2013; Lambek 2013; Rose and Novas 2005.

31 I am extremely grateful to an anonymous reviewer for suggesting some of the formulations in the above two paragraphs.

1 "Donating Blood for 26 Years," *The Star*, April 2, 2008.

2 "Donating Blood for 26 Years."

3 "Chief Inspector among 300 Blood Donors," *The Star*, May 27, 2008.

4 "Drive Nets 43 Pints of Blood," *The Star*, March 11, 2008.

5 "Hashers Donate Blood," *The Star*, June 28, 2008.

6 "Hashers Donate Blood."

7 "Members Who Have Paid Can Vote Elsewhere," *The Star*, June 2, 2008.

8 "Transplant Touches Hearts," *The Star*, October 6, 2007, accessed October 31, 2007, https://www.thestar.com.my/news/nation/2007/10/06/transplant-touches -hearts/.

9 "Happy to Be Home Again," *The Star*, February 6, 2008.

10 "A 'New' Birthday for Hui Yi," *The Star*, March 5, 2008.

11 "Paying Tribute to Muslim Couple," *The Star*, March 5, 2008.

12 "Muslims to Be Included in Organ Law," *New Straits Times*, January 23, 2008.

13 "Reward Organ Donors and Give Their Families Incentives," *The Star*, May 5, 2008; "Attracting Donors," *The Star*, July 20, 2008.

14 "Fulfilling Daughter's Wish," *The Star*, May 7, 2008.

15 "Parents Refuse to Honour Children's Pledge after Deaths," *The Star*, May 15, 2008.

CHAPTER ONE. BLOOD DONATION

1 See also Laqueur (1999) and the introduction to this book for discussion of the "gift relationship" in Titmuss's work. My thanks to Geoffrey Hughes for his articulation of the tension between different kinds of gifts that blood donation encompasses.

2 The pervasive association between blood and life (see Kuriyama 2002) is explored elsewhere in this book: see the introduction, chapter 4, and the conclusion.

3 See also Adams, Erwin, and Le 2010 for a subtle analysis of the tensions and reworkings of ideas and practices of suitable compensation for "patriotic" blood donation in China in the wake of contamination scandals.

4 I am grateful to Laura Bear for encouraging me to think about different forms of gendered labor here.

5 I am grateful to Catherine Allerton for this suggestion and to an anonymous reviewer for encouraging me to push further the ideas in this paragraph. Allerton observes that blood banks in Malaysia accept blood from at least some noncitizens (personal communication).

1 "Sign Up for 080808 Wedding," *The Star*, May 30, 2008.
2 "Full Load," *The Star*, June 19, 2008.
3 "Ways to Beat Rising Healthcare Costs," *The Star*, June 10, 2008.
4 "More Converging on Govt Hospitals," *The Star*, July 3, 2008.
5 "Man Gets Nod from Wives and Court to Marry a Fourth," *The Star*, June 10, 2008.
6 "Family Not Taken with Mr Wonderful," *The Star*, June 8, 2008.

CHAPTER TWO. LAB SPACES AND PEOPLE

1 These authors note, however, that the statistics do not capture the extent of women's participation in the informal economy. They also observe that women's participation in the formal sector rose sharply after 1970 but has leveled off since 1990 (tan and Ng 2014, 350). See also Jamilah 1994 on women's rising participation rates in education in Malaysia. Ariffin notes that while "overtly there seems to be no sex discrimination in Malaysian society . . . there are still certain fields of education and employment that women would not be encouraged to venture into" (1994, 70).

2 The economic plans were instituted in 1957 but were intensified with the Second Malaysia Plan of 1971–75, after ethnic riots in Kuala Lumpur in 1969 and as part of a "New Economic Policy" from 1971 to 1990 designed to address Malay economic grievances, mainly through encouraging Malay urbanization and entry into entrepreneurships and managerial positions (see Means 1991; Milne and Mauzy 1999; Yeoh 2014a).

3 For discussions of Malaysian politics under Mahathir, see Crouch 1996; Hilley 2001; Means 1991; Milne and Mauzy 1999. See also Khoo 1995; Mahathir 1970, 1986, 1993, for accounts of Mahathir's vision of "Asian values." For a recent survey of these developments see Yeoh 2014a.

4 It is likely, because of both employment practices in the public sector and the preferences of employees, that the proportion of Malay staff would have been higher in Penang's public hospital than in the private hospitals where I carried out research.

5 For discussions of changing educational policies in Malaysia, see Brown 2007; Lee 2014; Neville 1998; Selvaratnam 1988.

6 See Ong 2016 for a discussion of how an "ethnic heuristic" linking biomarkers, genetic defects, and ethnic difference is deployed in different registers in biomedical genetic research on cancer in Singapore and China.

7 I am grateful to an anonymous reviewer for encouraging me to think further about the fishponds.

1 For a full account of Anwar Ibrahim's trial from 2010 to 2012, the events preceding it, his acquittal at that trial, the subsequent appeal by the prosecution, and Anwar's eventual conviction and sentence to five years' imprisonment for sodomy in 2015 by the Federal Court, see Trowell 2015.

2 Under the Malaysian Penal Code, "sodomy" is a punishable offense, a statute originating from British colonial rule that has not been subsequently repealed (Kirby 2015).

3 "Anwar: Proof on Najib Soon," *The Star*, July 4, 2008.

4 "'Anwar Was Not Stripped Naked' HKL Director: His Decency Was Not Violated," *The Star*, July 20, 2008.

5 The status of DNA samples of both Anwar Ibrahim and Mohd Saiful Bukhari, submitted by the prosecution, was central and highly contested in the subsequent trial in 2010–12. Anwar had continued to refuse to give DNA samples, but police retrieved items from his police cell without his consent and submitted these for DNA analysis. The defense disputed the admissibility of these and also questioned the integrity of samples obtained from Mohd Saiful's rectum, in part because of the length of time that had elapsed between the alleged assault and when the samples were taken. Questions were also raised about the subsequent handling and storage of Mohd Saiful's DNA samples, their possible degradation, and the broken "chain of custody" of these exhibits (see Trowell 2015, 120–35).

6 "'I Am PM of All Races,' Abdullah: It Is My Duty to Be Honest and Fair to Everyone," *The Star*, February 28, 2008.

7 "Passing the Baton," *The Star*, February 24, 2008.

8 "M'sians against Street Demos," *The Star*, February 13, 2008.

9 Martin Vengadesan, "Truth and Reconciliation," *The Star*, May 11, 2008.

10 There has been extensive academic discussion and analysis of the 2008 election results in Malaysia and their implications; see, for example, Chin and Wong 2009; Maznah 2008; Lian and Appudurai 2011; O'Shannassay 2009; Ooi, Saravanamuttu, and Lee 2008; Pepinsky 2009; Weiss 2009. On the importance of new media in Malaysia see Weiss 2013.

11 While the subsequent trial hinged on evidence from (highly contested) DNA samples, the prominence of blood in the newspaper reports of the early stages of these events is suggestive. Franklin (2013) discusses the resilience and deep embeddedness of blood idioms in the face of new discourses of geneticization, which she attributes to the long history of the former in relation to the latter.

CHAPTER THREE. THE WORK OF THE LABS

1 I am grateful to Ayala Emmet for suggesting this term.
2 It was clear from memos on the lab notice boards that the hospital management was concerned to bring down the financial costs of medical treatment following needle prick injuries.
3 The identifying number of the hospital and the donor as well as the computer check digit given here have been changed.
4 I thank an anonymous reviewer for suggesting these comparisons.
5 I am grateful to Ian Harper for suggesting the term "rehumanizing" and underlining its importance to lab work.

PUBLIC LIFE OF BLOOD IV. MEDICAL, SUPERNATURAL, AND MORAL MATTERS

1 Siegel notes, for example, the "power of that dead body such that its force always exceeds the power of murderers" (1998, 114), a depiction that is reminiscent of stories I was told in the 1980s in Langkawi.
2 "All Abuzz over Oily Man," *The Star*, February 1, 2008.
3 "Father Wants to Sell Kidney," *The Star*, July 4, 2008.
4 "Growing Threat of Hepatitis C," *The Star*, June 25, 2008.
5 "Kidney Transplants Suspended," *The Star*, April 1, 2008.
6 "HIV+ Blood Donor Jailed," *The Star*, May 16, 2008.
7 "Girl Makes Medical History," *The Star*, January 25, 2008.
8 "Group Stole 1,000 Body Parts," *The Star*, February 1, 2008.
9 "Designer Babies Unacceptable," *The Star*, June 18, 2008.
10 "Ministry Wants Women to Take Precaution," *The Star*, June 1, 2008.
11 "A Test for You," *The Star*, March 9, 2008.
12 Milton Lum, "Hospital Charges and Fee Splitting," *The Star*, May 18, 2008.
13 "We Are JCI Accredited! Joint Commission International. Meeting International Safety and Quality Healthcare Standards," *The Star*, June 13, 2008.

CHAPTER FOUR. GHOSTS, FOOD, AND RELATEDNESS

1 I am particularly grateful to Gillian Feeley-Harnik for helping to draw out these ideas.
2 Such self-consciously "modern" venues were sometimes favored for lunch and had the advantage of not catering exclusively to any particular ethnic food preferences.

3 See Furth 1999 for an examination of postpartum ideas and practices in Chinese medical history.

4 See Kuriyama 2002 on layers of the body and treatment in classical Chinese medicine. In Penang I was told by practitioners of Chinese medicine that practices in Malaysia and Singapore are very similar to each other, and both were more traditional than Chinese medicine in China, which is more Western-influenced. On traditional medicine in contemporary China see Sivin 1987.

5 In his evocation of *A New Criminal Type in Jakarta*, James Siegel also notes how ghosts are associated with particular sites, especially those of death (1998, 88).

6 For a full account of ghosts and spirit medium practices in the context of Chinese popular religion in Penang, and for a more historical framing of these practices, see DeBernardi 2004, 2006.

7 I am grateful to Tom Gibson for encouraging me to think through these ideas.

8 As Thomas Laqueur has remarked, however, "There are no ambiguities in Titmuss" (1999, 3).

CONCLUSION

1 I am grateful to Rayna Rapp for suggesting "velocity" of blood.

REFERENCES

Adams, Vincanne, Kathleen Erwin, and Phuoc V. Le. 2010. "Governing through Blood: Biology, Donation, and Exchange in Urban China." In *Asian Biotech: Ethics and Communities of Fate*, edited by Aihwa Ong and Nancy N. Chen, 167–89. Durham, NC: Duke University Press.

Allers, Charles. 2013. *The Evolution of a Muslim Democrat: The Life of Malaysia's Anwar Ibrahim*. New York: Peter Lang.

Allerton, Catherine. 2013. *Potent Landscapes: Place and Mobility in Eastern Indonesia*. Honolulu: University of Hawai'i Press.

Amrith, Megha. 2013. "Encountering Asia: Narratives of Filipino Medical Workers on Caring for Other Asians." *Critical Asian Studies* 45 (2): 231–54.

Amrith, Sunil S. 2013. *Crossing the Bay of Bengal: The Furies of Nature and the Fortunes of Migrants*. Cambridge, MA: Harvard University Press.

Anagnost, Ann. 2006. "Strange Circulations: The Blood Economy in Rural China." *Economy and Society* 35 (4): 509–29.

Anidjar, Gil. 2014. *Blood: A Critique of Christianity*. New York: Columbia University Press.

Appadurai, Arjun. 1981. "Gastro-Politics in Hindu South Asia." *American Ethnologist* 8 (3): 494–511.

Appadurai, Arjun, ed. 1986. *The Social Life of Things: Commodities in Cultural Perspective*. Cambridge: Cambridge University Press.

Banerjee, Dwaipayan. 2014. "Writing the Disaster: Substance Activism after Bhopal." In *South Asian Tissue Economies*, edited by Jacob Copeman, 36–48. London: Routledge.

Barad, Karen. 2003. "Posthumanist Performativity: Toward an Understanding of How Matter Comes to Matter." *Signs: Journal of Women in Culture and Society* 28 (3): 801–31.

Baud, Jean-Pierre. 2011. "La nature juridique du sang." *Terrain* 56: 90–105.

Bautista, Julius. 2012a. "Preface: Motion, Devotion, and Materiality in Southeast Asia." In *The Spirit of Things: Materiality and Religious Diversity in Southeast*

Asia, edited by Julius Batista, vii–x. Ithaca, NY: Cornell Southeast Asia Program Publications.

Bautista, Julius, ed. 2012b. *The Spirit of Things: Materiality and Religious Diversity in Southeast Asia*. Ithaca, NY: Cornell Southeast Asia Program Publications.

Baxstrom, Richard. 2008. *Houses in Motion: The Experience of Place and the Problem of Belief in Urban Malaysia*. Stanford, CA: Stanford University Press.

Baxstrom, Richard. 2014. "Can the Law Do Justice? Everyday Ethics and the Transformation of Urban Life in Kuala Lumpur." In *The Other Kuala Lumpur: Living in the Shadows of a Globalising Southeast Asian City*, edited by Yeoh Seng Guan, 41–71. London: Routledge.

Bayly, Christopher, and Tim Harper. 2005. *Forgotten Armies: Britain's Asian Empire and the War with Japan*. London: Penguin.

Bayly, Christopher, and Tim Harper. 2007. *Forgotten Wars: The End of Britain's Asian Empire*. London: Penguin.

Bear, Laura. 2007. "Ruins and Ghosts: The Domestic Uncanny and the Materialization of Anglo-Indian Genealogies in Kharagpur." In *Ghosts of Memory: Essays on Remembrance and Relatedness*, edited by Janet Carsten, 36–57. Malden, MA: Blackwell.

Bear, Laura. 2013. "'This Body Is Our Body': *Vishwakarma Puja*, the Social Debts of Kinship, and Theologies of Materiality in a Neoliberal Shipyard." In *Vital Relations: Modernity and the Persistent Life of Kinship*, edited by Susan McKinnon and Fenella Cannell, 155–77. Santa Fe, NM: SAR Press.

Bear, Laura. 2014. "Doubt, Conflict and Mediation: An Anthropology of Modern Time." *Journal of the Royal Anthropological Institute*, n.s., 20 (S1): 3–30.

Berg, Marc, and Annemarie Mol, eds. 1998. *Differences in Medicine: Unraveling Practices, Techniques, and Bodies*. Durham, NC: Duke University Press.

Bildhauer, Bettina. 2013. "Medieval European Conceptions of Blood: Truth and Human Integrity." In *Blood Will Out: Essays on Liquid Transfers and Flows*, edited by Janet Carsten, 56–75. Malden, MA: Wiley-Blackwell.

Bloch, Maurice. 1973. "The Long Term and the Short Term: The Economic and Political Significance of the Morality of Kinship." In *The Character of Kinship*, edited by Jack Goody, 75–88. Cambridge: Cambridge University Press.

Bloch, Maurice. 1977. "The Past and the Present in the Present." *Man*, n.s., 12: 278–92.

Bloch, Maurice, and Jonathan Parry. 1989. "Introduction: Money and the Morality of Exchange." In *Money and the Morality of Exchange*, edited by Jonathan Parry and Maurice Bloch, 1–32. Cambridge: Cambridge University Press.

Bonney, Rollin. 1971. *Kedah, 1771–1821: The Search for Security and Independence*. Kuala Lumpur: Oxford University Press.

Born, Georgina. 2015. "Making Time: Temporality, History, and the Cultural Object." *New Literary History* 46 (3): 361–86.

Bowker, Geoffrey C., and Susan Leigh Star. 1999. *Sorting Things Out: Classification and Its Consequences*. Cambridge, MA: MIT Press.

Brown, Graham K. 2007. "Making Ethnic Citizens: The Policy and Practice of Education in Malaysia." *International Journal of Educational Development* 27 (3): 318–30.

Bynum, Caroline Walker. 2007. *Wonderful Blood: Theology and Practice in Late Medieval Northern Germany and Beyond*. Philadelphia: University of Pennsylvania Press.

Cannell, Fenella. 1999. *Power and Intimacy in the Christian Philippines*. Cambridge: Cambridge University Press.

Cannell, Fenella. 2013. "The Re-enchantment of Kinship?" In *Vital Relations: Modernity and the Persistent Life of Kinship*, edited by Susan McKinnon and Fenella Cannell, 217–40. Santa Fe, NM: SAR Press.

Carsten, Janet. 1995a. "The Politics of Forgetting: Migration, Kinship and Memory on the Periphery of the Southeast Asian State." *Journal of the Royal Anthropological Institute*, n.s., 1 (2): 317–35.

Carsten, Janet. 1995b. "The Substance of Kinship and the Heat of the Hearth: Feeding, Personhood, and Relatedness among Malays of Pulau Langkawi." *American Ethnologist* 22 (2): 223–41.

Carsten, Janet. 1997. *The Heat of the Hearth: The Process of Kinship in a Malay Fishing Community*. Oxford: Clarendon.

Carsten, Janet. 2004. *After Kinship*. Cambridge: Cambridge University Press.

Carsten, Janet. 2011. "Substance and Relationality: Blood in Contexts." *Annual Review of Anthropology* 40: 19–35.

Carsten, Janet. 2013. "Introduction: Blood Will Out." In *Blood Will Out: Essays on Liquid Transfers and Flows*, edited by Janet Carsten, 1–23. Malden, MA: Wiley-Blackwell.

Carsten, Janet, and Stephen Hugh-Jones, eds. 1995. *About the House: Lévi-Strauss and Beyond*. Cambridge: Cambridge University Press.

Chaveau, Sophie. 2011. "Du don à l'industrie: La transfusion sanguine en France depuis les années 1940." *Terrain* 56: 74–89.

Chee Heng Leng, Andrea Whittaker, and Heong Hong Por. 2017. "Medical Travel Facilitators, Private Hospitals and International Medical Travel in Assemblage." *Asia Pacific Viewpoint* 58 (2): 242–54.

Chin, James, and Wong Chin Huat. 2009. "Malaysia's Electoral Upheaval." *Journal of Democracy* 20 (3): 71–85.

Cohen, Lawrence. 2005. "Operability, Bioavailability, and Exception." In *Global Assemblages: Technology, Politics, and Ethics as Anthropological Problems*, edited by Aihwa Ong and Stephen J. Collier, 79–90. Malden, MA: Blackwell.

Copeman, Jacob. 2004. "Blood Will Have Blood: A Study in Indian Political Ritual." *Social Analysis* 48 (3): 126–48.

Copeman, Jacob. 2005. "Veinglory: Exploring Processes of Blood Transfer between Persons." *Journal of the Royal Anthropological Institute*, n.s., 11 (3): 465–85.

Copeman, Jacob. 2008. "Violence, Non-violence, and Blood Donation in India." *Journal of the Royal Anthropological Institute*, n.s., 14 (2): 278–96.

Copeman, Jacob. 2009a. "Gathering Points: Blood Donation and the Scenography of 'National Integration' in India." *Body and Society* 15 (2): 71–99.

Copeman, Jacob. 2009b. "Introduction: Blood Donation, Bioeconomy, Culture." *Body and Society* 15 (2): 1–28.

Copeman, Jacob. 2009c. *Veins of Devotion: Blood Donation and Religious Experience in North India.* New Brunswick, NJ: Rutgers University Press.

Copeman, Jacob. 2013. "The Art of Bleeding: Memory, Martyrdom, and Portraits in Blood." In *Blood Will Out: Essays on Liquid Transfers and Flows*, edited by Janet Carsten, 147–69. Malden, MA: Wiley-Blackwell.

Copeman, Jacob. 2014. "Introduction: South Asian Tissue Economies." In *South Asian Tissue Economies*, edited by Jacob Copeman, 1–19. London: Routledge.

Crouch, Harold. 1996. *Government and Society in Malaysia.* Ithaca, NY: Cornell University Press.

Daniel, E. Valentine. 1984. *Fluid Signs: Being a Person the Tamil Way.* Berkeley: University of California Press.

Das, Veena. 2000. "The Practice of Organ Transplants: Networks, Documents, Translations." In *Living and Working with the New Medical Technologies: Intersections of Inquiry*, edited by Margaret Lock, Allan Young, and Alberto Cambrosio, 263–87. Cambridge: Cambridge University Press.

DeBernardi, Jean. 2004. *Rites of Belonging: Memory, Modernity, and Identity in a Malaysian Chinese Community.* Stanford, CA: Stanford University Press.

DeBernardi, Jean. 2006. *The Way That Lives in the Heart: Chinese Popular Religion and Spirit Mediums in Penang, Malaysia.* Stanford, CA: Stanford University Press.

Douglas, Mary. 1966. *Purity and Danger: An Analysis of Concepts of Pollution and Taboo.* London: Routledge and Kegan Paul.

Douglas, Mary. (1970) 2003. *Natural Symbols.* Abingdon, UK: Routledge.

Edwards, Jeanette. 2000. *Born and Bred: Idioms of Kinship and New Reproductive Technologies in England.* Oxford: Oxford University Press.

Erwin, Kathleen. 2006. "The Circulatory System: Blood, Procurement, AIDS, and the Social Body in China." *Medical Anthropology Quarterly* 20 (2): 139–59.

Faubion, James, ed. 2001. *The Ethics of Kinship: Ethnographic Enquiries.* Lanham, MD: Rowman and Littlefield.

Feeley-Harnik, Gillian. 1995. "Religion and Food: An Anthropological Perspective." *Journal of the American Academy of Religion* 63 (3): 565–82.

Feeley-Harnik, Gillian. 2013. "Placing the Dead: Kinship, Slavery, and Free Labor in Pre– and Post–Civil War America." In *Vital Relations: Modernity and the Persistent Life of Kinship*, edited by Susan McKinnon and Fenella Cannell, 179–216. Santa Fe, NM: SAR Press.

Feldman, Eric A., and Ronald Bayer, eds. 1999. *Blood Feuds: AIDS, Blood, and the Politics of Medical Disaster.* Oxford: Oxford University Press.

Filippucci, Paola, Joost Fontein, John Harries, and Cara Krmpotich. 2012. "Encountering the Past: Unearthing Remnants of Humans in Archaeology and Anthropology." In *Archaeology and Anthropology: Past, Present and Future*, edited by David Shankland, 197–218. London: Berg.

Fontein, Joost, and John Harries. 2013. "Editorial: The Vitality and Efficacy of Human Substances." *Critical African Studies* 5 (3): 115–26.

Fortes, Meyer. 1969. *Kinship and the Social Order.* London: Routledge and Kegan Paul.

Foucault, Michel. (1978) 1979. *History of Sexuality.* Vol. 1, *The Will to Knowledge*, translated by Robert Hurley. London: Penguin.

Foucault, Michel. 1985. *The History of Sexuality.* Vol. 2, *The Use of Pleasure*, translated by Robert Hurley. New York: Pantheon.

Foucault, Michel. 1991. "Governmentality." In *The Foucault Effect*, edited by Graham Burchell, Colin Gordon, and Peter Miller, 87–105. London: Harvester Wheatsheaf.

Francis, Gavin. 2015. *Adventures in Human Being.* London: Profile Books.

Franklin, Sarah. 2013. "From Blood to Genes? Rethinking Consanguinity in the Context of Geneticisation." In *Blood and Kinship: Matter for Metaphor from Ancient Rome to the Present*, edited by Christopher H. Johnson, Bernhard Jussen, David Warren Sabean, and Simon Teuscher, 285–306. New York: Berghahn.

Fraser, Suzanne, and Kylie Valentine. 2006. "'Making Blood Flow': Materialising Blood in Body Modification Practice and Blood-Borne Virus Prevention." *Body and Society* 12 (1): 97–119.

Freud, Sigmund. (1919) 2003. "The Uncanny." In *The Uncanny*, translated by David McLintock, with an introduction by Hugh Haughton, 121–62. London: Penguin.

Frow, John. 1997. *Time and Commodity Culture: Essays in Cultural Theory and Postmodernity.* Oxford: Clarendon.

Furth, Charlotte. 1999. *A Flourishing Yin: Gender in China's Medical History, 960–1665.* Berkeley: University of California Press.

Gentner, Dedre, Brian Bowdle, Phillip Wolff, and Consuelo Boronat. 2001. "Metaphor Is Like Analogy." In *The Analogical Mind: Perspectives from Cognitive*

Science, edited by Dedre Gentner, Keith J. Holyoak, and Biocho N. Kokinov, 199–253. Cambridge, MA: MIT Press.

Goh Beng-Lan. 2002. *Modern Dreams: An Enquiry into Power, Cultural Production, and the Cityscape in Contemporary Urban Penang, Malaysia*. Ithaca, NY: Cornell Southeast Asia Program Publications.

Gupta, Akhil. 1995. "Blurred Boundaries: The Discourse of Corruption, the Culture of Politics, and the Imagined State." *American Ethnologist* 22 (2): 375–402.

Harper, Tim N. 1999. *The End of Empire and the Making of Malaya*. Cambridge: Cambridge University Press.

Healy, Kieran. 2006. *Last Best Gifts: Altruism and the Market for Human Blood and Organs*. Chicago: University of Chicago Press.

Hilley, John. 2001. *Malaysia: Mahathirism, Hegemony and the New Opposition*. London: Zed Books.

Hirschmann, Charles. 1986. "The Making of Race in Colonial Malaya: Political Economy and Racial Ideology." *Sociological Forum* 1 (2): 330–61.

Hirschmann, Charles. 1987. "The Meaning and Measurement of Ethnicity in Malaysia: An Analysis of Census Classifications." *Journal of Asian Studies* 46 (3): 555–82.

Hoek, Lotte. 2014. "Blood Splattered Bengal: The Spectacular Spurting of Blood of the Bangladeshi Cinema." In *South Asian Tissue Economies*, edited by Jacob Copeman, 20–35. London: Routledge.

Ho Engseng. 2006. *The Graves of Tarim: Genealogy and Mobility across the Indian Ocean*. Berkeley: University of California Press.

Holland, Dorothy, and Jean Lave, eds. 2001. *History in Person: Enduring Struggles, Contentious Practice, Intimate Identities*. Santa Fe, NM: SAR Press.

Holst, Frederik. 2012. *Ethnicization and Identity Construction in Malaysia*. Abingdon, UK: Routledge.

Hugh-Jones, Stephen. 2011. "Analyses de sang." *Terrain* 56: 4–21.

Ingold, Tim. 2007. *Lines: A Brief History*. Oxford: Routledge.

Jamilah Ariffin. 1994. *Women and Development in Malaysia*. Rev. ed. Kelana Jaya, Malaysia: Pelanduk.

Jenkins, Gwynn. 2008. *Contested Space: Cultural Heritage and Identity Reconstructions. Conservation Strategies within a Developing Asian City*. Zurich: Lit Verlag.

Johnson, Christopher H., Bernhard Jussen, David Warren Sabean, and Simon Teuscher, eds. 2013. *Blood and Kinship: Matter for Metaphor from Ancient Rome to the Present*. New York: Berghahn.

Kahn, Joel. 2006. *Other Malays: Nationalism and Cosmopolitanism in the Modern Malay World*. Singapore: Singapore University Press.

Khoo Boo Teik. 1995. *Paradoxes of Mahathirism: An Intellectual Biography of Mahathir Mohamad.* Kuala Lumpur: Oxford University Press.

Khoo Kay Kim. 1972. *The Western Malay States, 1850–1873: The Effects of Commercial Development on Malay Politics.* Kuala Lumpur: Oxford University Press.

Khoo Su Nin. 1993. *Streets of George Town, Penang: An Illustrated Guide to Penang's City Streets and Historic Attractions.* Penang: Janus.

Kirby, Michael. 2015. Foreword to *The Prosecution of Anwar Ibrahim: The Final Play,* by Mark Trowell, 9–24. Singapore: Marshall Cavendish.

Krementsov, Nikolai. 2011. *A Martian Stranded on Earth: Alexander Bogdanov, Blood Transfusions, and Proletarian Science.* Chicago: University of Chicago Press.

Kua Kia Soong. 2007. *May 13: Declassified Documents on the Malaysian Riots of 1969.* Petaling Jaya, Malaysia: SUARAM.

Kuriyama, Shigehisa. 2002. *The Expressiveness of the Body and the Divergence of Greek and Chinese Medicine.* New York: Zone.

Kwon, Heonik. 2008. *Ghosts of War in Vietnam.* Cambridge: Cambridge University Press.

Lambek, Michael. 2011. "Kinship as Gift and Theft: Acts of Succession in Mayotte and Israel." *American Ethnologist* 38 (1): 2–16.

Lambek, Michael. 2013. "Kinship, Modernity, and the Immodern." In *Vital Relations: Modernity and the Persistent Life of Kinship,* edited by Susan McKinnon and Fenella Cannell, 241–60. Santa Fe, NM: SAR Press.

Lambert, Helen. 2000. "Sentiment and Substance in North Indian Forms of Relatedness." In *Cultures of Relatedness: New Approaches to the Study of Kinship,* edited by Janet Carsten, 73–89. Cambridge: Cambridge University Press.

Laqueur, Thomas. 1999. "Pint for Pint." *London Review of Books,* October 14, 3–7.

Latour, Bruno. 1983. "Give Me a Laboratory and I Will Raise the World." In *Science Observed: Perspectives on the Social Study of Science,* edited by Karin D. Knorr-Cetina and Michael Mulkay, 141–70. London: Sage.

Latour, Bruno. 1993. *We Have Never Been Modern.* Translated by Catherine Porter. London: Harvester Wheatsheaf.

Lederer, Susan E. 2008. *Flesh and Blood: Organ Transplantation and Blood Transfusion in Twentieth-Century America.* New York: Oxford University Press.

Lederer, Susan E. 2013. "Bloodlines: Blood Types, Identity, and Association in Twentieth-Century America." In *Blood Will Out: Essays on Liquid Transfers and Flows,* edited by Janet Carsten, 117–28. Malden, MA: Wiley-Blackwell.

Lee, Molly N. N. 2014. "Educational Reforms in Malaysia: Towards Equity, Quality and Efficiency." In *Routledge Handbook of Contemporary Malaysia,* edited by Meredith L. Weiss, 302–11. London: Routledge.

Lewis, Su Lin. 2016. *Cities in Motion: Urban Life and Cosmopolitanism in Southeast Asia.* Cambridge: Cambridge University Press.

Lian Kwen Fee and Jayanath Appudurai. 2011. "Race, Class and Politics in Peninsular Malaysia: The General Election of 2008." *Asian Studies Review* 35 (1): 63–82.

Lock, Margaret, Julia Freeman, Rosemary Sharples, and Stephanie Lloyd. 2006. "When It Runs in the Family: Putting Susceptibility Genes in Perspective." *Public Understanding of Science* 15: 277–300.

Lubis, Abdur-Razzaq. 2009. "Perceptions of Penang: Views from Across the Straits." In *Penang and Its Region: The Story of an Asian Entrepôt,* edited by Yeoh Seng Guan, Loh Wei Leng, Khoo Salma Nasution, and Neil Khor, 150–79. Singapore: NUS Press.

Mahani Musa. 1999. "Malays and the Red and White Flag Societies in Penang, 1830s–1920s." *Journal of the Malaysian Branch of the Royal Asiatic Society* 72 (2): 151–82.

Mahathir Mohamad. 1970. *The Malay Dilemma.* Singapore: Times Books International.

Mahathir Mohamad. 1986. *The Challenge.* Selangor, Malaysia: Pelanduk.

Mahathir Mohamad. 1993. "Views and Thoughts of the Prime Minister of Malaysia." In *Malaysia's Vision 2020: Understanding the Concept, Implications and Challenges,* edited by Ahmad Sarji Abdul Hamid. Petaling Jaya, Malaysia: Pelanduk.

Manickam, Sandra Khor. 2015. *Taming the Wild: Aborigines and Racial Knowledge in Colonial Malaya.* Singapore: NUS Press.

Marriott, McKim. 1976. "Hindu Transactions: Diversity without Dualism." In *Transaction and Meaning: Directions in the Anthropology of Exchange and Symbolic Behavior,* edited by Bruce Kapferer, 109–42. Philadelphia: Institute for the Study of Human Issues.

Martin, Emily. 1998. "Anthropology and the Cultural Study of Science." In "Anthropological Approaches in Science and Technology Studies," special issue, *Science, Technology and Human Values* 23 (1): 24–44.

Martin, Emily. 2013. "Blood and the Brain." In *Blood Will Out: Essays on Liquid Transfers and Flows,* edited by Janet Carsten, 170–82. Malden, MA: Wiley-Blackwell.

Mayblin, Maya. 2013. "The Way Blood Flows: The Sacrificial Value of Intravenous Drip Use in Northeast Brazil." In *Blood Will Out: Essays on Liquid Transfers and Flows,* edited by Janet Carsten, 42–55. Malden, MA: Wiley-Blackwell.

Maznah Mohamad. 2008. "Malaysia—Democracy and the End of Ethnic Politics?" *Australian Journal of International Affairs* 62 (4): 441–59.

Maznah Mohamad. 2010. "The Ascendance of Bureaucratic Islam and the Secularization of the Sharia in Malaysia." *Pacific Affairs* 83 (3): 505–24.

Maznah Mohamad. 2013. "Legal-Bureaucratic Islam in Malaysia: Homogenizing and Ring-Fencing the Muslim Subject." In *Encountering Islam: The Politics of*

Religious Identities in Southeast Asia, edited by Hui Yew-Foong, 103–32. Singapore: Institute of Southeast Asian Studies.

McKinley, Robert. 2001. "The Philosophy of Kinship: A Reply to Schneider's *Critique of the Study of Kinship.*" In *The Cultural Analysis of Kinship: The Legacy of David M. Schneider,* edited by Richard Feinberg and Martin Oppenheimer, 131–67. Urbana: University of Illinois Press.

McKinnon, Susan, and Fenella Cannell. 2013. "The Difference Kinship Makes." In *Vital Relations: Modernity and the Persistent Life of Kinship,* edited by Susan McKinnon and Fenella Cannell, 3–38. Santa Fe, NM: SAR Press.

Means, Gordon P. 1976. *Malaysian Politics.* 2nd ed. London: Hodder and Stoughton.

Means, Gordon P. 1991. *Malaysian Politics: The Second Generation.* Singapore: Oxford University Press.

Miller, Daniel. 2005. "Materiality: An Introduction." In *Materiality,* edited by Daniel Miller, 1–50. Durham, NC: Duke University Press.

Milne, Robert S., and Diane K. Mauzy. 1999. *Malaysian Politics under Mahathir.* London: Routledge.

Milner, Anthony. 2011. *The Malays.* Oxford: Wiley-Blackwell.

Milner, Anthony, and Helen Ting. 2014. "Race and Its Competing Paradigms: A Historical Review." In *Transforming Malaysia: Dominant and Competing Paradigms,* edited by Anthony Milner, Abdul Rahman Embong, and Tham Siew Yean, 18–58. Singapore: Institute of Southeast Asian Studies.

Mol, Annemarie. 1998. "Missing Links, Making Links: The Performance of Some Atheroscleroses." In *Differences in Medicine: Unraveling Practices, Techniques, and Bodies,* edited by Marc Berg and Annemarie Mol, 144–65. Durham, NC: Duke University Press.

Mol, Annemarie. 2002. *The Body Multiple: Ontology in Medical Practice.* Durham, NC: Duke University Press.

Mol, Annemarie, and Marc Berg. 1998. "Differences in Medicine: An Introduction." In *Differences in Medicine: Unraveling Practices, Techniques, and Bodies,* edited by Marc Berg and Annemarie Mol, 1–12. Durham, NC: Duke University Press.

Mollona, Massimiliano. 2005. "Factory, Family and Neighbourhood: The Political Economy of Informal Labour in Sheffield." *Journal of the Royal Anthropological Institute,* n.s., 11 (3): 527–48.

Morgan, Lewis Henry. 1871. *Systems of Consanguinity and Affinity of the Human Family.* Washington, DC: Smithsonian Institution Press.

Mumtaz, Zubia, and Adrienne Levay. 2014. "Forbidden Exchanges and Gender: Implications for Blood Donation during a Maternal Health Emergency in Punjab, Pakistan." In *South Asian Tissue Economies,* edited by Jacob Copeman, 66–80. London: Routledge.

Neville, Warwick. 1998. "Restructuring Tertiary Education in Malaysia: The Nature and Implications of Policy Changes." *Higher Education Policy* 11 (4): 257–79.

Nirenberg, David. 2009. "Was There Race before Modernity? The Example of 'Jewish' Blood in Late Medieval Spain." In *The Origins of Racism in the West*, edited by Miriam Eliav-Feldon, Benjamin Isaac, and Joseph Ziegler, 232–65. Cambridge: Cambridge University Press.

Nonini, Donald M. 2015. *"Getting By": Class and State Formation among Chinese in Malaysia*. Ithaca, NY: Cornell University Press.

Ong, Aihwa. (1987) 2010. *Spirits of Resistance and Capitalist Discipline: Factory Women in Malaysia*. 2nd ed. Introduction by Carla Freeman. Albany: State University of New York.

Ong, Aihwa. 2010a. "Introduction: An Analytics of Biotechnology at Multiple Scales." In *Asian Biotech: Ethics and Communities of Fate*, edited by Aihwa Ong and Nancy N. Chen, 1–51. Durham, NC: Duke University Press.

Ong, Aihwa. 2010b. "Lifelines: The Ethics of Blood Banking for Family and Beyond." In *Asian Biotech: Ethics and Communities of Fate*, edited by Aihwa Ong and Nancy N. Chen, 190–214. Durham, NC: Duke University Press.

Ong, Aihwa. 2016. *Fungible Life: Experiment in the Asian City of Life*. Durham, NC: Duke University Press.

Ong, Aihwa, and Nancy N. Chen, eds. 2010. *Asian Biotech: Ethics and Communities of Fate*. Durham, NC: Duke University Press.

Ooi Kee Beng, Johan Saravanamuttu, and Lee Hock Guan. 2008. *March 8: Eclipsing May 13*. Singapore: Institute of Southeast Asian Studies.

O'Shannassay, Michael. 2009. "Beyond the Barisan Nasional? A Gramscian Perspective of the 2008 Malaysian General Election." *Contemporary Southeast Asia: A Journal of International and Strategic Affairs* 31 (1): 88–109.

Peletz, Michael G. 2002. *Islamic Modern: Religious Courts and Cultural Politics in Malaysia*. Princeton, NJ: Princeton University Press.

Pepinsky, Thomas P. 2009. "The 2008 Malaysian Election: An End to Ethnic Politics?" *Journal of East Asian Studies* 9 (1): 87–120.

Pfeffer, Naomi, and Sophie Laws. 2006. "'It's Only a Blood Test': What People Know and Think about Venupuncture and Blood." *Social Science and Medicine* 62 (12): 3011–23.

Pinney, Christopher. 2005. "Things Happen, or From Which Moment Does That Object Come?" In *Materiality*, edited by Daniel Miller, 256–72. Durham, NC: Duke University Press.

Porqueres i Gené, Enric. 2007. "Kinship Language and the Dynamics of Race: The Basque Case." In *Race, Ethnicity and Nation: Perspectives from Kinship and Genetics*, edited by Peter Wade, 125–44. Oxford: Berghahn.

Rabinow, Paul. 1999. *French DNA: Trouble in Purgatory*. Chicago: University of Chicago Press.

Rapp, Rayna. 1999. *Testing Women, Testing the Fetus: The Social Impact of Amniocentesis in America*. New York: Routledge.

Roff, William R. 1994. *The Origins of Malay Nationalism*. Kuala Lumpur: Oxford University Press.

Rose, Nikolas, and Carlos Novas. 2005. "Biological Citizenship." In *Global Assemblages: Technology, Politics, and Ethics as Anthropological Problems*, edited by Aihwa Ong and Stephen J. Collier, 439–63. Malden, MA: Blackwell.

Sabean, David Warren, and Simon Teuscher. 2013. Introduction to *Blood and Kinship: Matter for Metaphor from Ancient Rome to the Present*, edited by Christopher H. Johnson, Bernhard Jussen, David Warren Sabean, and Simon Teuscher, 1–17. New York: Berghahn.

Sanabria, Emilia. 2009. "Alleviative Bleeding: Bloodletting, Menstruation and the Politics of Ignorance in a Brazilian Blood Donation Centre." *Body and Society* 15 (2): 123–44.

Schneider, David M. (1968) 1980. *American Kinship: A Cultural Account*. Chicago: University of Chicago Press.

Schneider, David M. 1984. *A Critique of the Study of Kinship*. Ann Arbor: University of Michigan Press.

Seeman, Don. 1999. "'One People, One Blood': Public Health, Political Violence, and HIV in an Ethiopian-Israeli Setting." *Culture, Medicine and Psychiatry* 23 (2): 159–95.

Seeman, Don. 2010. *One People, One Blood: Ethiopian-Israelis and the Return to Judaism*. New Brunswick, NJ: Rutgers University Press.

Selvaratnam, Viswanathan. 1988. "Ethnicity, Inequality, and Higher Education in Malaysia." *Comparative Education Review* 32 (2): 173–96.

Shamsul, A. B. 1996. "Debating about Identity in Malaysia: A Discourse Analysis." *Tonan Ajia Kenkyu* 34 (3): 566–600.

Shamsul, A. B. 1998. "Ethnicity, Class, Culture or Identity? Competing Paradigms in Malaysian Studies." *Akademika* 53: 33–59.

Shamsul, A. B. 2001. "The Redefinition of Politics and the Transformation of Malaysian Pluralism." In *The Politics of Multiculturalism: Pluralism and Citizenship in Malaysia, Singapore, and Indonesia*, edited by Robert W. Hefner, 204–26. Honolulu: University of Hawai'i Press.

Shamsul, A. B., and S. M. Athi. 2014. "Ethnicity and Identity Formation: Colonial Knowledge, Colonial Structures and Transition." In *Routledge Handbook of Contemporary Malaysia*, edited by Meredith L. Weiss, 267–78. London: Routledge.

Shao Jing. 2006. "Fluid Labor and Blood Money: The Economy of HIV/AIDS in Rural Central China." *Cultural Anthropology* 21 (4): 535–69.

Shao Jing and Mary Scoggin. 2009. "Solidarity and Distinction in Blood: Contamination, Morality and Variability." *Body and Society* 15 (2): 29–50.

Shever, Elana. 2013. "'I Am a Petroleum Product': Making Kinship Work on the Patagonian Frontier." In *Vital Relations: Modernity and the Persistent Life of Kinship*, edited by Susan McKinnon and Fenella Cannell, 85–107. Santa Fe, NM: SAR Press.

Siegel, James T. 1998. *A New Criminal Type in Jakarta: Counter-Revolution Today.* Durham, NC: Duke University Press.

Simpson, Bob. 2004. "Impossible Gifts: Bodies, Buddhism and Bioethics in Contemporary Sri Lanka." *Journal of the Royal Anthropological Institute*, n.s., 10 (4): 839–59.

Simpson, Bob. 2009. "Please Give a Drop of Blood: Blood Donation, Conflict and the Haemato-Global Assemblage in Contemporary Sri Lanka." *Body and Society* 15 (2): 101–22.

Simpson, Bob. 2011. "Blood Rhetorics: Donor Campaigns and Their Publics in Contemporary Sri Lanka." *Ethnos* 76 (2): 254–75.

Singleton, Vicky. 1998. "Stabilizing Instabilities: The Role of the Laboratory in the United Kingdom Cervical Screening Programme." In *Differences in Medicine: Unraveling Practices, Techniques, and Bodies*, edited by Marc Berg and Annemarie Mol, 86–104. Durham, NC: Duke University Press.

Sivin, Nathan. 1987. *Traditional Medicine in Contemporary China. Science, Medicine and Technology in East Asia* 2. Ann Arbor: Center for Chinese Studies, University of Michigan.

Ssorin-Chaikov, Nikolai. 2006. "On Heterochrony: Birthday Gifts to Stalin, 1949." *Journal of the Royal Anthropological Institute*, n.s., 12 (2): 355–75.

Stafford, Charles. 2000. *Separation and Reunion in Modern China.* Cambridge: Cambridge University Press.

Star, Susan Leigh. 1989. "The Structure of Ill-Structured Solutions: Boundary Objects and Distributed Artificial Intelligence." In *Distributed Artificial Intelligence*, vol. 2, edited by Les Gasser and Michael N. Huhns, 37–54. Menlo Park, CA: Morgan Kauffmann.

Star, Susan Leigh, and James R. Griesemer. 1989. "Institutional Ecology, 'Translations' and Boundary Objects: Amateurs and Professionals in Berkeley's Museum of Vertebrate Zoology, 1907–39." *Social Studies of Science* 19 (3): 387–420.

Starr, David. 1998. *Blood: An Epic History of Medicine and Commerce.* London: Warner Books.

Stoler, A. 1992. "Sexual Affronts and Racial Frontiers: European Identities and the Cultural Politics of Exclusions in Colonial Southeast Asia." *Comparative Studies in Society and History* 34 (3): 514–51.

Stoler, A. 1997. "On Political and Psychological Essentialisms." *Ethos* 25 (1): 101–6.

Street, Alice. 2009. "Failed Recipients: Extracting Blood in a Papua New Guinean Hospital." *Body and Society* 15 (2): 193–216.

Strong, Thomas. 2009. "Vital Publics of Pure Blood." *Body and Society* 15 (2): 169–91.

Tagliacozzo, Eric. 2013. *The Longest Journey: Southeast Asians and the Pilgrimage to Mecca*. Oxford: Oxford University Press.

tan beng hui and Cecilia Ng. 2014. "Filling in the Gaps: The Pursuit of Gender Equality in Malaysia." In *Routledge Handbook of Contemporary Malaysia*, edited by Meredith L. Weiss, 347–60. London: Routledge.

Tan Liok Ee. 2002. "Chinese Education in Malaysia Today." In *Ethnic Chinese in Singapore and Malaysia: A Dialogue between Tradition and Modernity*, edited by Leo Suryadinata, 155–71. Singapore: Times Academic Press.

Tan Liok Ee. 2009. "Conjunctures, Confluences, Contestations: A Perspective on Penang History." In *Penang and Its Region: The Story of an Asian Entrepôt*, edited by Yeoh Seng Guan, Loh Wei Leng, Khoo Salma Nasution, and Neil Khor, 7–29. Singapore: NUS Press.

Taylor, Christopher C. 1992. *Milk, Honey, and Money: Changing Concepts in Rwandan Healing*. Washington, DC: Smithsonian Institution Press.

Thompson, Eric C. 2003. "Malay Male Migrants: Negotiating Contested Identities in Malaysia." *American Ethnologist* 30 (3): 418–38.

Thompson, Eric C. 2007. *Unsettling Absences: Urbanism in Rural Malaysia*. Singapore: NUS Press.

Thompson, Stuart. 1988. "Death, Food and Fertility." In *Death Ritual in Late Imperial and Modern China*, edited by James L. Watson and Evelyn S. Rawski, 71–108. Berkeley: University of California Press.

Titmuss, Richard. (1970) 1997. *The Gift Relationship: From Human Blood to Social Policy*. Rev. ed. Edited by Ann Oakley and John Ashton. New York: New Press.

Trautmann, Thomas R. 1987. *Lewis Henry Morgan and the Invention of Kinship*. Berkeley: University of California Press.

Trowell, Mark. 2015. *The Prosecution of Anwar Ibrahim: The Final Play*. Singapore: Marshall Cavendish.

Turnbull, C. M. 2009. "Penang's Changing Role in the Straits Settlements, 1826–1946." In *Penang and Its Region: The Story of an Asian Entrepôt*, edited by Yeoh Seng Guan, Loh Wei Leng, Khoo Salma Nasution, and Neil Khor, 30–53. Singapore: NUS Press.

Turner, Victor. 1967. *The Forest of Symbols: Aspects of Ndembu Ritual*. Ithaca, NY: Cornell University Press.

Tutton, Richard. 2002. "Gift Relationships in Genetics Research." *Science as Culture* 11 (4): 523–42.

Valentine, Kylie. 2005. "Citizenship, Identity, Blood Donation." *Body and Society* 11 (2): 113–28.

Verdery, Katherine. 1999. *The Political Lives of Dead Bodies: Reburial and Postsocialist Change*. New York: Columbia University Press.

Wade, Peter. 1993. "'Race,' Nature and Culture." *Man*, n.s., 28 (1): 1–18.

Wade, Peter. 2002. *Race, Nature and Culture: An Anthropological Perspective*. London: Pluto.

Wade, Peter, ed. 2007. *Race, Ethnicity and Nation: Perspectives from Kinship and Genetics*. Oxford: Berghahn.

Waldby, Catherine, and Robert Mitchell. 2006. *Tissue Economies: Blood, Organs, and Cell Lines in Late Capitalism*. Durham, NC: Duke University Press.

Warner, Marina. 2016. "Those Brogues." *London Review of Books*, October 6, 29–32, http://www.lrb.co.uk/v38/n19/marina-warner/those-brogues.

Weiss, Meredith L. 2009. "Edging Towards a New Politics in Malaysia: Civil Society at the Gate?" *Asian Survey* 49 (5): 741–58.

Weiss, Meredith L. 2013. "Parsing the Power of 'New Media' in Malaysia." *Journal of Contemporary Asia* 43 (4): 591–612.

Weston, Kath. 2001. "Kinship, Controversy, and the Sharing of Substance: The Race/Class Politics of Blood Transfusion." In *Relative Values: Reconfiguring Kinship Studies*, edited by Sarah Franklin and Susan McKinnon, 147–74. Durham, NC: Duke University Press.

Weston, Kath. 2013. "Lifeblood, Liquidity, and Cash Transfusions: Beyond Metaphor in the Cultural Study of Finance." In *Blood Will Out: Essays on Liquid Transfers and Flows*, edited by Janet Carsten, 24–41. Malden, MA: Wiley-Blackwell.

Whitfield, Nicholas. 2013. "Who Is My Stranger? Origins of the Gift in Wartime London. 1939–45." In *Blood Will Out: Essays on Liquid Transfers and Flows*, edited by Janet Carsten, 94–116. Malden, MA: Wiley-Blackwell.

Whittaker, Andrea, Chee Heng Leng, and Por Heong Hong. 2017. "Regional Circuits of International Medical Travel: Prescriptions of Trust, Cultural Affinity and History." *Asia Pacific Viewpoint* 58 (2): 136–47.

Williams, Brackette F. 1995. "Classification Systems Revisited: Kinship, Caste, Race, and Nationality as the Flow of Blood and the Spread of Rights." In *Naturalizing Power: Essays in Feminist Cultural Analysis*, edited by Sylvia Yanagisako and Carol Delaney, 201–38. New York: Routledge.

Yanagisako, Sylvia J. 2002. *Producing Culture and Capital: Family Firms in Italy*. Princeton, NJ: Princeton University Press.

Yanagisako, Sylvia J. 2013. "Transnational Family Capitalism: Producing 'Made in Italy' in China." In *Vital Relations: Modernity and the Persistent Life of Kinship*, edited by Susan McKinnon and Fenella Cannell, 63–84. Santa Fe, NM: SAR Press.

Yanagisako, Sylvia J., and Carol Delaney. 1995. "Naturalizing Power." In *Natural-izing Power: Essays in Feminist Cultural Analysis*, edited by Sylvia Yanagisako and Carol Delaney, 1–22. New York: Routledge.

Yeoh Seng Guan. 2012. "Holy Water and Material Religion in a Pilgrimage Shrine in Malaysia." In *The Spirit of Things: Materiality and Religious Diversity in Southeast Asia*, edited by Julius Batista, 79–94. Ithaca, NY: Cornell Southeast Asia Program Publications.

Yeoh Seng Guan. 2014a. "The Great Transformation: Urbanisation and Urbanism in Malaysia." In *Routledge Handbook of Contemporary Malaysia*, edited by Meredith L. Weiss, 249–59. London: Routledge.

Yeoh Seng Guan. 2014b. "Introduction: The World Class City and Subaltern Kuala Lumpur." In *The Other Kuala Lumpur: Living in the Shadows of a Globalising Southeast Asian City*, edited by Yeoh Seng Guan, 1–21. London: Routledge.

Yeoh Seng Guan, ed. 2014c. *The Other Kuala Lumpur: Living in the Shadows of a Globalising Southeast Asian City*. Oxford: Routledge.

Yeoh Seng Guan. 2019. "Domesticating Anthropology in West Malaysia." In *South-east Asian Anthropologies: National Traditions and Transnational Practices*, edited by Eric C. Thompson and Vineeta Sinha, 141–68. Singapore: National University of Press.

Yeoh Seng Guan, Loh Wei Leng, Khoo Salma Nasution, and Neil Khor, eds. 2009. *Penang and Its Region: The Story of an Asian Entrepôt*. Singapore: NUS Press.

Zawawi Ibrahim and Ahmad Fauzi Abdul Hamid. 2017. "The Governance of Religious Diversity in Malaysia: Islam in a Secular State or Secularism in an Islamic State?" In *The Problem of Religious Diversity: European Chal-lenges, Asian Approaches*, edited by Anna Triandafyllidou and Tariq Modood, 169–203. Edinburgh: Edinburgh University Press.

blood groups: blood donation and, 14; group O, 5; Malay ideas of, on Langkawi, 4–5; rare, 64–65, 146; Rhesus–negative, 67, 104; testing for, 135–38. *See also* domaining

blood screening. *See* blood donation; hepatitis; HIV; laboratory work; lupus; syphilis

blood symbolism, 4–16, 30–34, 200–208; politics and, 116–24, 210n11; temporality of, 9–15. *See also* citizenship; ethnicity; health; kinship; morality; nationhood; naturalization

Born, Georgina, 209n9

boundary objects: blood as, 71; blood donor enrollment forms and, 63, 71–72; concept of, 8–9, 12–13. *See also* domaining; rehumanization

Bowker, Geoffrey, 8–9, 12–13, 63, 71–72, 205

Cannell, Fenella, 4, 31–32, 201

Chen, Nancy N., 14

childbirth. *See* blood: childbirth; Malay: childbirth

Chinese community, 17–19; Baba-Nyonya (Peranankan) or Chinese-Malay community, 17

Chinese medicine, 30, 173, 183–86, 209n3, 216n4

citizenship, 31; blood and, 72–74, 212n5 (chapter 1). *See also* nationhood

clinical pathology labs. *See* laboratories

Copeman, Jacob, 10

Das, Veena, 72

death: blood and, 7, 193; life and, 3–4; in the Philippines, 4. *See also* ghosts

DeBernardi, Jean, 21, 188

detachment: laboratory work and, 127–28, 141–42, 150, 155–56. *See*

also domaining; naturalization; objectification; purification; rehumanization

dialysis, 41, 123

DNA, 116, 118, 214n5, 214n11

domaining, 6, 14, 208; blood and, 11, 30; boundary practices, 70, 112, 148, 155, 167–68, 193–99; modernity and, 32–34, 156, 208. *See also* blood donor booklets; blood donor enrollment forms; blood groups; boundary objects; domestication; detachment; laboratory work: labeling; naturalization; objectification; purification; rehumanization

domestication, 176; laboratories and, 79–81, 112, 156–57, 167–68, 194–98. *See also* rehumanization

economies of care, 69, 72

education: schooling, 17, 19; tertiary sector, 19, 96–98. *See also* ethnicity; laboratory workers

Edwards, Jeanette, 150

ethnicity: blood and, 104, 203–4; blood transfusion and, 153–54; development and, 96; economy and, 20–21; education and, 17, 97–98; local understandings of, 21–22, 101–4; national politics and, 18–20, 22, 120–22; in Penang, 16–22; "race" and, 18–19, 66–68; religion and, 16–17, 19–20, 97. *See also* blood donor enrollment forms; blood donors; laboratory workers; organ donation

fate, 109, 110. *See also* luck

Feeley-Harnik, Gillian, 31–32, 215n1 (chapter 4)

Fontein, Joost, 11–12

food, 169–71; blood donation and, 49–50, 56, 59–60; commensality,

200–201, 203–4; in laboratories, 87.
See also laboratory workers: commensality among; Malay: food

Foucault, Michel, 31

Franklin, Sarah, 15, 214n11

Freud, Sigmund, 186

Furth, Charlotte, 216n3

gender. *See* blood donors; laboratories;
laboratory workers

Gentner, Dedre, 13

George Town, 16, 18, 20, 21

Gerakan (Malaysian People's Movement Party), 20

ghosts, 8, 30, 165–66, 186–91; blood and,
158–59, 188, 191; distribution of, 187;
in Indonesia, 158–59, 188; thieves and,
158–59, 188; in Vietnam, 3–4. *See also*
orang minyak; spirits; uncanny, the;
vampire spirits

Gibson, Thomas, 216n7

gifts: blood donation as gift, 14, 45–46,
59–62, 72, 197–98, 204, 212n1
(chapter 1); gifts given to blood
donors, 28, 43, 45, 49, 54, 57, 59–62.
See also food; money

Gupta, Akhil, 211n29

Harper, Ian, 215n5 (chapter 3)

Harries, John, 11–12

Harvey, William, 9

health: blood and, 29; blood donation
and, 57–59

hepatitis, 71, 135, 146, 160

HIV, 70, 104, 118, 131, 160–61; blood
screening and, 69, 135, 146, 154

hospitals: fieldwork in, 23–25; in Penang, 20–21; private, 59–65; public,
59–65. *See also* blood donation;
ghosts; laboratories; laboratory
work; medical costs; organ donation; trust

Indian community, 18–20; Indian
Muslims, 17

Islam. *See* blood; education: schooling;
nationhood; organ donation

Jamilah Ariffin, 213n1 (chapter 2)

Jawi Peranakan community, 17–19

kinship: blood and, 4, 10, 15; blood
donation and, 36, 51–57; blood transfusion and, 153–54; idioms used in
laboratories, 139–40; laboratory work
and, 152–54, 167–68; Malay ideas
of, 5, 175–76; modernity and, 31–32,
201–2, 207–8. *See also* blood donors:
kinship; laboratory workers: sociality
among

Kuriyama, Shigehisa, 3, 7, 34, 209n1,
216n4

Kwon, Heonik, 3–4, 189

laboratories, 80–115, 200–201; as field
site, 23–24; gender in, 89; spatiality
of, 80–91, 111–12, 114–15, 193–95; as
workspaces, 28, 79–80. *See also* domestication; food; ghosts; hospitals;
kinship; laboratory work; laboratory
workers; morality

laboratory work, 29, 33–34, 81–82,
125–57, 203; blood processing, 28–29,
46; hygiene and, 87–88, 131–34;
labeling, 142–48; modernity and, 168;
taking blood, 129–34; testing blood,
134–40. *See also* detachment; kinship;
luck; objectification; purification;
rehumanization; risk; trust

laboratory workers, 7, 15, 23; commensality among, 169–71, 175–76; education and, 91, 94–99, 113; ethics and,
176–82; ethnicity and, 97–99, 101–5,
114, 175–76, 195; gender and, 93, 95,
99–101, 136; knowledge flows among,

laboratory workers (cont.)
182–86; personality types and, 105–11, 113; sociality among, 29–30, 89–91, 127–31, 154–57, 172–99, 203; sociology of, 28, 91–115; training and, 125–26, 128–29, 133–34, 156

Langkawi, 4, 17, 22, 123, 158, 176

Laqueur, Thomas, 212n1 (chapter 1), 216n8

Latour, Bruno, 81, 114–15, 168, 197

Laws, Sophie, 131

life: blood and, 7, 191–93, 205–7; death and, 3–4. *See also* animation; vitality

luck, 75, 109; in laboratory work, 133. *See also* fate

lupus, 135, 180

Mahathir Mohamad, 19, 27, 96–98, 113, 122, 213n3 (chapter 2)

Malay: blood, Malay ideas about, 154, 185; blood groups, Malay ideas of, on Langkawi, 4–5; childbirth, Malay ideas about, 173–74; ethnic category of, 21; food, Malay ideas about, 175–76, 185; kinship, Malay ideas about, 5, 175–76; Malay identity and Islam, 19, 211n24

Malayan Chinese Association/Malaysian Chinese Association (MCA), 20, 36, 122

Malayan Indian Congress/Malaysian Indian Congress (MIC), 20, 122

Malay community, 17–19; government policies and, 97–98, 213n2

Malay medicine, 173, 183, 184

Martin, Emily, 10, 193

Mayblin, Maya, 9, 10

Maznah Mohamad, 211n24, 214n10

McKinnon, Susan, 31–32, 201

medical costs, 76, 162–63; hospital charges, 52, 61–62, 161–62

medical tourism, 20, 23

Mitchell, Robert, 14

modernity, 73, 93. *See also under* domaining; kinship; laboratory work

Mohd Saiful Bukhari, 117, 214n5

Mol, Annemarie, 29, 150, 155

money, 8. *See also* gifts; medical costs

morality: blood and, 27–28, 131, 158–64, 202–3, 204–5; blood donation and, 44, 70–73; laboratories and, 155–56. *See also* Anwar Ibrahim: blood sample case; gifts

Morgan, Lewis Henry, 31–32, 207

Najib Tun Razak, 117, 122

nationhood: blood and, 37–42; Malay identity and Islam, 19, 211n24. *See also* citizenship

naturalization, 9, 31–33; blood and, 11–13, 15, 73, 205–7. *See also* domaining

newspapers: consumption of news, 75–78, 89–90; as ethnographic resource, 25, 26. *See also* blood donation: newspaper coverage of; organ donation: newspaper coverage of

Nonini, Donald, 21

objectification: blood and, 11, 65; information and, 140–42; labeling and, 148; samples and, 29, 127–29. *See also* detachment; domaining; naturalization; purification; rehumanization

Ong, Aiwa, 14, 22, 159, 213n6 (chapter 1)

orang minyak (oily man), 159. *See also* ghosts; spirits; uncanny, the; vampire spirits

organ donation: donor shortages, 40–42; ethnicity and, 37–42, 67–68; heart transplants, 37–40; Islam and, 41, 68, 154; newspaper coverage of, 77–78, 160; statistics of, 41–42

Partai Ra'ayat/Parti Rakyat, 20, 116–17

Parti se Islam Malaysia (PAS), 122

Printed and bound by CPI Group (UK) Ltd, Croydon, CR0 4YY

27/10/2024

14580225-0005